Generic Drugs

A Consumer's Self-Defense Guide

Clifford L. Nilsen

iUniverse, Inc.
Bloomington

Generic Drugs
A Consumer's Self-Defense Guide

iUniverse books may be ordered through booksellers or by contacting:

iUniverse
1663 Liberty Drive
Bloomington, IN 47403
www.iuniverse.com
1-800-Authors (1-800-288-4677)

ISBN: 978-1-4502-8346-5 (pbk)
ISBN: 978-1-4502-8408-0 (cloth)
ISBN: 978-1-4502-8409-7 (ebk)

Library of Congress Control Number: 2010919342

Printed in the United States of America

iUniverse rev. date: 1/26/12

Contents

Introduction..vii

Chapter One—The Basics... 1

Chapter Two—Truth Or Consequences 9

Chapter Three—Drug Approvals and the Generic World 66

Chapter Four—Real Generic Stories—Nilsen's Believe It
                    Or Not... 105

Chapter Five—Active Pharmaceutical Ingredients................ 112

Chapter Six—Self Defense.. 120

Appendix I.. 145

Appendix II.. 189

Introduction

Imagine the horror as you rush your infant child to the hospital emergency room. "Doctor, what's wrong?" "We can't be sure miss, but it looks like some kind of poisoning". After a short time, the Doctor comes back out to tell the hysterical mother "I'm sorry, but your baby died". What happened? Upon investigation, it was determined that the mother had given the baby a generic brand of infant ear drops for an ear ache. It turns out that the ear drops contained glycerin as a main ingredient, glycerin from China that was contaminated with anti-freeze. How could that possibly happen? This story is fictional, but glycerin from China contaminated with anti-freeze is real. How can we as consumers avoid buying contaminated or substandard drug products? Do you know if the products sitting in your medicine chest or kitchen cabinets are safe to use? How can you be sure?

This book uncovers and documents questionable manufacturing practices used by drug companies, mostly generic companies that could have serious health consequences for American consumers who purchase the drugs produced by those companies. No one wants to use drug products that are contaminated with dangerous chemicals, foreign matter such as metal and glass, or harmful bacteria, or wants to purchase and use drugs that are mislabeled or have the wrong strength, or that have been made using shoddy manufacturing procedures in dirty equipment by untrained workers. Yet, these things are commonplace, particularly with over the counter (OTC) generic drugs. Chapter 1 introduces the reader to drug company basics and Food and Drug Administration (FDA) inspections. In Chapter 2, "Truth or Consequences", a comparison is made between what drug companies are supposed to do and what they actually do. Specific examples of violations are shown to provide the reader with an appreciation of how badly things are often screwed up in drug manufacturing. Chapter 3, although necessarily a bit technical in spots, walks you through the process of how a new drug gets on the market and how a generic substitute gets approved. In order to understand the full impact of generic drug practices, it is useful, by contrast, to explain the complexity involved in a new drug approval. This chapter also reveals why generics may not be equivalent to brand name drugs. Finally, the dirty little secrets of the generic OTC world are exposed, showing you the risks and potential dangers of using these products. Chapter 4 recounts actual personal experiences with a number of at-risk companies, while Chapter 5 presents a look at the dangers of active ingredients, particularly materials imported from countries like China and India. Finally, Chapter 6, "Self Defense" describes the step-by step procedures you need to protect yourselves from buying or using potentially dangerous generic drug products.

This book gives you the information and tools necessary to protect you and your family from using questionable or potentially hazardous drug products. Russian roulette should not be the game of choice when purchasing drug products.

DISCLAIMER:
While the written content of this work is believed to be free of spelling and grammatical errors, FDA reports and website reprints and excerpts may not be. It is beyond the scope of this book for the author to correct or alter these items.

CHAPTER ONE
THE BASICS

Before diving into generic drugs in detail, a short introduction to the United States drug industry is in order. A drug company is any company that manufactures, holds, distributes packages or tests drug products. By Finished Drug Products, we mean what you, the consumer, buy at your drug store or supermarket, either by prescription or over the counter.

Rules & Regulations:

Drug manufacturers in virtually every country of the world come under the jurisdiction of a regulatory agency of one kind or another. For example, in Europe it's the European Medicines Agency (EMEA), in Canada it's Health Canada, in Australia it's the Therapeutic Goods Administration (TGA), and here in the United States, it's the United States Food and Drug Administration (FDA). A law known as The United States Federal Food, Drug and Cosmetic Act, defines the requirements for the manufacture, holding and distribution of drug products in the United States. It is often referred to as simply "The Act".

Additionally, there is a body of work, known as the Code of Federal Regulations, based upon "The Act", that govern the "rules of the road" for most Federal agency regulations such as EPA, OSHA, Social Security, and of course, FDA. The Code of Federal Regulations contains many volumes, each of which is divided into many titles. Title 21, Parts 210 and 211, derived from "The Act", describes the rules of the road for manufacturing human drugs. Title 21, part 211, designated 21 CFR 211, is entitled "Current Good Manufacturing Practice for Finished Pharmaceuticals", more commonly referred to as simply cGMPs. Throughout the rest of this book, since Current Good Manufacturing Practices are the rules and regulations for drug manufacturers, they will be referred to as simply "GMPs". FDA inspects drug companies to make sure that they are following GMPs, which are legally binding.

In addition to GMPs, FDA has published a myriad of "Guidances for Industry", that attempt to provide a more expanded view of GMPs, and which attempt to reflect current FDA thinking on compliance issues. There are about 30 categories, each containing many individual guidances. These guidances are not legally binding, as are the GMPs, but in reality, they may as well be. The confusion is mind-boggling.

Ready for more?—In addition to GMPs and FDA Guidances, there is an additional set of guidances issued by the International Conference on Harmonisation or ICH. The ICH guidances are an attempt to standardize drug regulations and procedures between the United States and other countries.

Now the real fun begins. Regulations such as the GMPs are what are known as performance standards, that is they tell you what must be accomplished, but not how to do it. This makes for very wide and varied opinions and philosophies on just what to do in order to be in compliance. GMP compliance is, or should be, of paramount importance to drug companies, consumers and to the FDA, the body responsible for assuring compliance through inspection of drug manufacturers.

When it comes to compliance there are basically three kinds of drug companies.

- The ones who understand and actually comply with GMPs. These companies operate in responsible manner, producing drugs that are safe, effective and consistently reliable.
- Those who want and try to comply, but lack a thorough enough understanding of the how to correctly implement

2

GMPs, such that they receive numerous deficiencies during FDA inspections and wind up finding themselves in hot water, or even boiling water. These companies are often referred to as "honest but stupid"—often the result of poorly qualified personnel, under-staffing or ineffective training programs.

- Lastly, there are those who apparently don't care, or just don't get it and who are always in trouble. Unfortunately for American consumers, there are quite a few of these. Some are even guilty of willfully violating GMP regulations, resulting in potential serious threats to consumer health and safety. Scary, isn't it?, considering that there are many companies making the drugs that you or your children use, that are in violation of GMP requirements or worse, just plain willfully and sometimes criminally negligent.

In a later chapter of this book, I will name names and cite specific examples of drug GMP violations, including those that pose a major potential consumer health hazard. The list includes companies, some whose names are well-known, and who produce many household-name drug products that we have learned to trust over the years.

The Inspection Process:

Drug companies, when they first open their doors for business, must register with the FDA as a drug establishment, after which they are issued a registration number. The "Drug Establishment Registrations" must be renewed annually. There are several different types of registrations depending upon the nature of the drug establishment, i.e., manufacturer, packager, distributor or contract laboratory for example. Once a company has registered, they are on the FDA's radar and put on the regulatory inspection schedule.

By the way, anyone can start a drug company. Buy a bunch of manufacturing equipment cheap at auction (blenders, tablet presses, packaging and lab equipment, etc), set up in a garage or basement, and start manufacturing, so long as the operation is performed under GMP conditions, which is unlikely for what we will call "Garage Pharmaceuticals". The problem is that FDA probably won't get around to inspecting this firm for about two years, after which they will more than likely be shut down. But wait a minute; what about the drug products that have been pushed into the market place over those two years? Are they safe and effective? Maybe, maybe not. Unfortunately, there actually are some "Garage Pharmaceuticals" -type companies out there. Are you or your children using these drugs?—are they safe?—maybe, maybe not. Is there any way to be sure? Let's see.

FDA can initiate inspection of a drug establishment for any number of reasons.

Most common are-

- General inspections (a statutory bi-annual requirement)—this inspection is an audit conducted by FDA to assure compliance with GMP regulations. They look at a company's organization chart, training records, resumes of key personnel, manufacturing procedures and records, facility maintenance, cleaning, laboratory controls, packaging and labeling controls, validation, drug stability, complaints, recalls, failure investigations and more.

  NOTE: in FDA speak, FDA is referred to as "The Agency", and the company being inspected is referred to as "The Firm".

  FDA uses a snapshot approach, i.e., they randomly select several production batch records and follow them through the entire product life cycle which includes receipt of raw materials and packaging components, sampling and testing of these, quality review and release of these materials for use in manufacturing, manufacturing procedures, product yields, packaging and labeling and release of product to the market place. There is also a review of all laboratory testing, and adherence to internal procedures and quality systems. Additionally, if the firm used outside contractors to perform any of their manufacturing operations or portion thereof, those contractors become part of the firm's manufacturing process, and subsequently, the firm must demonstrate through a process of audit and vendor qualification, that those contractors are in compliance and are following GMP regulations as well. Examples are contract packagers and contract testing laboratories. FDA will also verify validation of manufacturing processes, laboratory test methods, cleaning procedures and certain computer software. If the snapshot looks "good", the inspection is a short one. However, if a pattern of violations is discovered that indicates systemic problems with the firm's GMP compliance, the inspection can get much more protracted and downright ugly.

At the end of the inspection, the FDA investigator will have a close-out meeting with management at which time an FDA Form 483, usually referred to as just " a 483", may be issued to the firm. If the inspection is favorable, i.e., no significant objectionable findings recorded, no 483 will be issued. On the other hand, if there are significant adverse findings, the FDA investigator will issue a 483. The 483 is nothing more than a list of observations. It lists objectionable findings, citing specific examples. The firm will usually respond within 15 days to the observations (See Chapter 2, "Truth or Consequences").

- Preapproval inspections (PAI)—Inspections performed before FDA approval of a new or generic drug for sale to consumers.
- Customer complaint or adverse medical event—a visit by FDA resulting from a customer complaint or because of a reported adverse drug reaction, such as a rash, headache, or other unexpected reaction to a drug product. FDA and company actions will depend upon the seriousness of the incident, ranging from a review of records to recall or seizure of product.

- Drug recall—The firm works with an FDA recall manager until the recall is finished and closed out.

  FDA usually shows up unannounced without prior warning. Upon arrival, they present their credentials (badge and ID) and then issue an FDA Form 482 to a responsible member of management. The 482 is the notice of inspection. Once it is issued, the inspection has begun. The most common type of inspection is the bi-annual, general GMP inspection. Companies with good track records will see FDA every two years. Others may see them more often.

  FDA now uses something that has taken hold in the past few years, called a systems-based inspection. Pharmaceutical company operations are divided into six main systems—production system, packaging and labeling system, materials system, laboratory controls system, facilities & equipment system and the most important, the quality system which is the cornerstone of pharmaceutical operations and which impacts and drives the other five systems. If the quality system is out of control or non-compliant, the whole operation is non-compliant.

  The actual United States Code of Federal Regulations, Title 21, Part 211, more commonly referred to as 21 CFR 211, "CURRENT GOOD MANUFACTURING PRACTICE FOR FINISHED PHARMACEUTICALS" can be found in Appendix I. The basic requirements for each system, i.e., what drug companies are supposed to do at minimum, and what FDA looks for, are as follows:

- Production Systems-

  Production systems include all aspects of manufacturing equipment including design, construction, cleaning and maintenance and control of equipment, plus manufacturing procedures including all documentation and other requirements needed to make a drug product under GMP conditions.

- Packaging & Labeling Systems-

  Control of packaging and labeling are of critical importance to not only the drug manufacturer, but to the consumer as well. Sloppy packaging or labeling practices could lead to mix-ups such as putting the wrong drug in a bottle, or mislabeling, either of which could have dire consequences.

  Proper controls involve having a system in place that absolutely prevents mix-ups or mislabeling. This, among other things, requires that every packaging component and label is accounted for.

- Materials System-

  This system includes control and handling of raw materials such as active and inactive ingredients, packaging components such as bottles, caps and cartons, plus warehousing, shipping and receiving.

- Laboratory Controls System-

  The quality control laboratory is the foundation upon which a drug company stands. Testing done by the Quality Control laboratory impacts every aspect of drug manufacturing. There must be a systems in place to ensure that all data produced are accurate and defensible. It is an immensely complex system that requires advanced skills and knowledge to manage properly. It is also the system that if deficient, can and often does, result in bad FDA inspections, Warning Letters or worse.

- Facilities and Equipment System-

  This system deals with the physical facility requirements ranging from design, ventilation, plumbing, lighting, sewerage and sanitation. Drug products need to be manufactured in a clean environment that is free of dirt, contamination and pests such as rodents, insect and birds.

- Quality Systems-

  The Quality System is the most important of all. It encircles all the other systems and is the one system that has "jurisdiction" over the others. The quality system is managed by a Quality Control Unit which has the sole authority to release or reject drug product. If the quality control unit says a batch is rejected, it is rejected. Even the company president or CEO cannot override that rejection, at least in theory. The quality control unit reviews every document that is created, changed or executed. This includes standard operating procedures, manufacturing procedures and documentation, cleaning procedures, laboratory test results, packaging records, validation work and more.

Text of regulations shown in Appendix I, illustrates the complexity of what is expected of drug companies for manufacture, holding and distribution of drug products in the United States. The GMP regulations are indeed complex. In addition, as previously mentioned, FDA has published a myriad of Guidances for Industry that further expand upon FDA thinking for execution of GMP regulations.

Do all companies follow GMPs correctly and conscientiously? Absolutely not! This is clearly evidenced by the number of serious inspection reports, Warning Letters, seizures, injunctions, consent decrees and debarments from the pharmaceutical industry.

Chapter 2, "Truth or Consequences", describes how things really work, and the price that is paid for non-compliance. Actual examples, naming names, are cited.

CHAPTER TWO
TRUTH OR CONSEQUENCES

Truth

Do you know where your drugs come from, how they were manufactured or whether or not they are safe, effective and contain the right amount of active ingredient? Before taking any drug yourself or giving it to one of your family members, you should know which drugs companies are reliable and which ones have a history of GMP problems. This information is public; later in this book we will spell out how to access it.

First of all, one needs to understand that GMPs, like most other standards such as OSHA, are performance standards. Performance standards, as previously mentioned, are regulations that spell out what you need to achieve, but not how to do it. For example, if I tell someone to do something—tell my son to clean his room for example, without any further input, he will clean it his way in a way that _he_ thinks is satisfactory. In other words, without specific guidance on how to clean the room, the outcome is unpredictable.

Drug companies face the same problem. Since they can choose how to achieve compliance with the regulations, the outcomes are unpredictable unless the firm has a solid understanding and control of the six systems described in Chapter One.

Firms need to have written procedures for everything they do in the form of some official written document such as a Standard Operating Procedure (SOP) or written test method. All of these documents must have been reviewed and approved by the Quality Control Unit, and most important, all written procedures must be followed <u>as written</u> each and every time. Consistent execution of written procedures is a key element of GMP compliance. When buying an OTC product or filling a prescription, you should not have to worry about whether or not the drug manufacturer is making your drug product the same way every time, and in line with all GMP regulations.

The burden of compliance rests with the drug manufacturer. Whenever a firm asks FDA "how am I supposed to do this", the answer will always be "you're supposed to know that". Since every company operates differently, individual drug company operating procedures also vary widely, which is fine so long as those procedures are effective in meeting cGMP requirements. Drug companies must interpret how to meet FDA expectations of compliance and therein lays the problem. These interpretations, even when firms are conscientiously trying their best, do not always hit the mark.

Drug companies carry a huge burden in their quest for good compliance. Some examples of basic expectations are as follows:

- Manufacturing processes need to be written and followed consistently, from dispensing of ingredients to packaging, labeling, testing and shipping.
- Manufacturing processes must be validated. *Note: Validation is the process of proving that something consistently works the way it's supposed to.*
- Cleaning procedures need to be written and followed consistently.
- Cleaning procedures must be validated.
- Laboratory test methods need to be written, followed consistently and validated.
- There has to be system of document control for issuing and revising documents.
- Certain computer systems need to be validated.

- Training must be given and documented for every operation.
- Effectiveness of training must be demonstrated and documented.
- Microbiological contamination must be controlled, particularly for water systems and sterile drug manufacturing.
- All documentation such as standard operating procedures, analytical test methods, manufacturing and packaging procedures, validation protocols and reports and quality reports, laboratory and manufacturing data, batch records, complaints and non-conformance investigations must be reviewed by the Quality Control Unit.

It is no surprise that drug companies often fail the test of FDA inspection. Those firms whose inspections go poorly consist of three basic types. The first is the company that tries to be compliant, but for some reason, perhaps understaffing, deficient training, or maybe even a lack of understanding of how to properly apply cGMP practices, still fails to make the grade. The second is the company that knows the regulations and has the resources to be GMP compliant, but who takes shortcuts and tries to get around the regulations for the sake of profit or convenience. The third type of company is one that frankly just doesn't give a shit and willfully ignores regulations to the point that consumer safety is compromised.

Are there many drug companies that are in one of these three categories?—absolutely. Are there many drug companies that are in the second or third category? You bet. Because the regulations (GMPs) are performance standards that allow for wide interpretation as to how to achieve those standards, individual concepts of how to comply, i.e., companies adapting the regulations to fit their individual business models, often leads to a conflict between what companies do and what FDA expects. FDA is always raising the bar often making it difficult for companies to stay in compliance or stay in tune with latest FDA thinking on GMP matters.

There are companies that get through FDA inspections with "flying colors" because upper management is committed to quality and compliance, and staffing levels allow for proper oversight of the six systems. Additionally, training and documentation are strong and personnel have the education, experience or training necessary to properly perform their assigned functions. The need for proper staffing and qualifications cannot be overstated. There have been instances where FDA has "leaned" on companies for inadequate staffing or competency. I personally, as a consultant, have witnessed FDA inspections that have resulted in terminations and rearrangement of personnel. These actions can range from firing of chemists or production operators to removal of a company president.

As previously mentioned, FDA investigators use a snapshot approach when doing GMP inspections. They first take a tour of areas such as the manufacturing facility, packaging areas, warehouse, pharmacy and laboratories. This part of the inspections is useful for getting an initial idea of how the company operates. The next step is to start reviewing documents. The investigator randomly selects several manufacturing batch records for review. The review will consist of verification that all written procedures were followed as written. This includes dispensing, actual manufacture of a drug product, packaging, label control, control of raw materials, testing of in-process and finished product samples, plus review of and approval of all documents related to the manufacture of that batch. FDA will also look at sequencing to be sure that all steps occurred in proper order. For example, was a raw material approved before it was used in a batch, or was the finished product tested after it was manufactured. If the sequencing is off, for example, a batch was tested before it was manufactured, the snapshot is dead. To cite an extreme example of sloppy record keeping, there was a firm back in the early 1990s that during an FDA inspection proved beyond a shadow of a doubt that a batch was destroyed five months before it was manufactured.

If the snapshot looks good, the inspection will be short one. On the other hand, if FDA finds one problem after another and starts to see systemic compliance problems, then the inspection will be long and unpleasant. What would otherwise be a three to five day inspection, may become a three or four week inspection. There have even been inspections that have gone on for months.

Since FDA inspections are generally unannounced, firms need to be in a good state of compliance at all times, which is what is expected. When purchasing a drug product at the local pharmacy, one shouldn't have to worry whether or not the manufacturer was in compliance the week they made that batch of drug. It is expected that all drug products are manufactured by companies that are in a good state of control at all times.

FDA investigators have the official title Consumer Safety Officer (CSO). They are charged with auditing drug companies for GMP compliance to make sure that drug products are manufactured that consistently meet standards of effectiveness, purity, identity and safety. FDA has a number of district offices across the United States that have inspectional jurisdiction over the firms in their district. FDA investigators are very well trained. They know what to look for, how to ask the right questions and are very good at unveiling problems, even ones the firm doesn't realize they have. They are experts at identifying non-conformance and fraud. When an inspection reveals that there are significant violations or fraud, investigators recommend courses of action to their district's compliance branch, whose actions will depend upon the severity of the violations. Drug manufacturing violations can range from minor infractions that are not a significant consumer risk to more serious problems that could result in people getting sick or worse yet, patient deaths.

Consequences:

There are several possible levels of FDA actions depending upon the inspection outcome.

These are:

- No 483—No action indicated. Company did well, can expect FDA back in two years for another routine inspection.
- 483 issued with minor observations—Voluntary action indicated. Firm must respond to the 483 observations within 15 days, providing a substantial plan for correcting

violations. A district's compliance officer handles this, and if satisfied with the response, will issue a letter indicating so. Firms can expect FDA back in about two years for another general GMP inspection, at which time the investigator will verify that violations from the previous inspection have been corrected.

- 483 issued with major observations—Involuntary action indicated. Firms must respond to 483 as stated above, however, because of serious violations, may be issued a Warning Letter.
- Warning Letters—A Warning Letter requires a remediation plan be submitted to FDA's compliance branch within 15 days of receipt. The plan may or may not be accepted by FDA. Once a plan is found to be acceptable, FDA will more than likely visit that company again more frequently, within six months for example. Once all corrections have been verified, the Warning Letter can be closed. Warning Letters are serious. They can damage a company's reputation, affect its ability to get government contracts, and impacts on their ability to get new drug approvals which is the lifeblood of many drug companies.
- Injunctions—If FDA feels that a firm's state of compliance and manufacturing procedures actually pose a threat to consumer safety, they may seek an injunction to stop the company from manufacturing and distributing drug products altogether.
- Consent decrees—For years, many companies would promise to fix objectionable observations, and then when re-inspected, would be cited once again for the same problems. In other words, talk is cheap, promises were not kept. The two most serious observations a firm can receive during an FDA inspection are not following their own written procedures and repeat violations from previous inspections. FDA has a trust but verify credo, i.e., they believe what you tell them, but they will verify it. FDA got tired of broken promises, so, in certain cases where a firm was made to cease operations, that firm had to enter into a consent decree

with FDA. A consent decree as once explained to me by the Director of an FDA District Office, is merely court-supervised corrective actions needed to return a firm to a state of control. Under a consent decree, a firm has to meet its corrective action obligations in order to get FDA clearance for resuming manufacturing and distribution of its drug products. A firm must hire a consultant to help them, and whose task it is, once corrections have been made, to recertify the company as GMP compliant. One the recertification is done, FDA is called back in for a re-inspection to verify that all remediations have been completed. Once the firm is back in operation, FDA will periodically inspect to verify that the company is maintaining suitable conformance to GMPs.

- Debarment—If a company president or other responsible person is involved in criminal activities such as fraud, they can be permanently or temporarily debarred from the industry, and if warranted, criminally prosecuted as well. FDA's website has a complete list of debarments.

Although many companies are in trouble, some of which are habitual offenders (real screw ups), FDA has also had its share of bad press. The great generic scandal of 1989 changed everything. During that time, some FDA officials were accepting bribes from certain companies to give them preferential treatment in the generic drug approval process. One company, Bolar Pharmaceuticals, actually put its own coating on brand name drugs and submitted them for approval as their own generic equivalent. How did they get caught, well surprise, surprise. FDA had a laboratory in Cincinnati with an instrument that could look through a tablet coating and see what is underneath. When the company's tablets were examined by the Cincinnati laboratory, the brand name was exposed underneath their tablet coating. The president of that company is on the debarment list. When investigations by Congress and by a few generic companies were over, several FDA officials, and some company officials, were criminally charged, with many resulting convictions. "Go to jail, do not pass go, do not collect $200.00". A new FDA commissioner, Dr. David Kessler, was appointed to run the agency and to help restore its reputation. Dr. Kessler, who is both a lawyer and a medical doctor, was an excellent commissioner. It was he who coined the phrase "trust but verify".

But why are there such problems with generic companies in particular? A major reason is that many generic drug companies are small, privately held or family-owned businesses with limited financial resources. As a result, when it comes to manufacturing operations and GMP compliance, shortcuts are often taken, and corners cut. These smaller companies depend heavily on stuff going out the door to maintain the cash flow needed to operate or to even survive. Rejecting batches or spending extra money is the last thing they need, so they often finagle their way around problems.

It is a basic GMP rule that if a batch is not made according to GMPs, even if it meets all of its specifications, it is considered adulterated (contaminated) and cannot be shipped to commerce. But this doesn't stop some firms who will come up with any lame excuse to ship the product anyway. It is also possible that they just don't understand the regulations. Also, if a batch fails to meet its specifications during the listed shelf life (not stable over time), it must be recalled. Rejections and recalls are expensive and as unwanted as the black plague.

Another problem is language. Many small companies, and some larger ones as well, are staffed mostly by employees from foreign countries like India, China, the Middle East or Latin America. It is often the case with foreign employees, who often work for peanuts, that English language skills are poor or marginal at best, resulting in communication problems that negatively impact manufacturing and laboratory operations. I have seen instances where entire departments within a company spoke virtually no English. How the hell can someone read procedures or be properly trained if they can't speak or understand English? How can they understand the true meaning and impact of GMP compliance? Being able to read and write English is a GMP requirement.

Another potential problem with foreign employees is that many are not U.S. citizens or don't have a Green Card. They hold visas that can tie them to one employer at whatever minimum pay is mandated for a particular job classification. For these folks to change jobs, they need to find a new employer who will transfer their visa which is both expensive and time consuming. If unemployed, many of these visa holders could be deported back to their country of origin. The result is a form of indentured servitude, which could be abused by a firm's management in the form of coercion to do what they're told, even if it violates regulations, for fear of losing their jobs and the resulting consequences thereof.

Many smaller generic companies have facilities that look like medieval dungeons, with poor lighting and environmental controls, not to mention lousy sanitation and other deficiencies such as poor microbiological control, contamination and mix ups.

Having run my own pharmaceutical contract laboratory for a number of years, with good FDA inspection results, including several PAI drug application approvals, I am proud to have been involved with an operation whose GMP compliance was of benchmark quality.

Let me clarify the term PAI. A PAI, as mentioned in Chapter One, is a pre-approval inspection. In the past, a company would submit an application for a generic drug approval, and based upon the scientific data submitted by the firm, FDA would approve the application. Then a funny thing happened. It was discovered that some companies lied. For example, a company might state in their application that they blend their drug in a 100 cubic foot blender and then compress tablets using a tablet press (brand is unimportant for this example), and then test the drug in their laboratory using a an instrument known as an HPLC. When the FDA inspects the company later on, guess what, they haven't got a 100 cubic foot blender, or even a tablet press. Not only that, there is no HPLC in the laboratory, or no laboratory at all. As a result, we now have pre-approval inspections (PAIs). These inspections are a final verification prior to approval of a generic drug application (or a new drug application for that matter). During the PAI, FDA will verify that the firm has all the equipment and systems mentioned in their drug application.

Now let's look at the other end of the spectrum, using an actual example. Back in the early 1990s there was a drug manufacturer in northern New Jersey (no longer in the drug business—name withheld for reasons of mercy) that should have been the poster boy for bad pharmaceutical manufacturing practices. They were a small, family-owned firm with very limited financial resources that ran hand to mouth. Their 50,000 square foot facility was a visual nightmare. This place made a medieval dungeon look like the Ritz-Carlton. The roof was shot and every time it rained, it also rained indoors in much of the facility. Laboratory chemists were actually issued umbrellas to avoid getting wet while working in the lab on rainy days. Laboratory data was often faked, manipulated or fabricated to make sure products "met" specifications. The packaging of drug products was conducted in an area that was a rat's nest of microbiological contamination. There was a garage door next to the packaging line that was left open to the outside. Employees did brake- jobs on their cars just outside that door. One of the owners brought his dog into work, and it wasn't unusual from time to time to see a huge 150 pound Newfoundland dog running around the facility. Products were stored for unacceptable lengths of time in drums, sometime that had been sitting around for years, and packaged when needed. Microbiological contamination in these products was controlled by throwing an arbitrary "handful" of preservative into the drum and hoping for the best.

What the hell was I doing there you might ask? This company had a long history of poor FDA inspections. As a consultant, I received a call for help after a very tough FDA investigator showed up and began a very intense and detailed inspection, with the intention of putting a chain on the front door. I was able to buy some time for the firm, but during the extension period, the company had a recall due to a dangerous gram negative bacteria that was discovered in a batch of anti-diarrhea medication that was shipped to nursing homes. That was the last straw, resulting in a seizure of the company's products by U.S. Marshalls and an injunction against the firm, after which the company discontinued manufacturing drug products—permanently.

The best way to illustrate the types of violations for which companies are cited is to present some actual examples of 483 observations. After many of these example observations, I will comment and pose a question for you, the reader, to think about. Please note that the examples presented throughout this book are public information, available to anyone on FDA's website or through the Freedom of Information Act (FOI). The first two sets are taken from inspections of two different generic drug manufacturers. The last set is from inspection of a name brand company whose products are household names, and which most of us have been using for many years. The brand name company is included here to show that it is not only generic firms that have GMP problems. The following are inspectional observations taken from actual FDA inspection reports:

Major generic drug company #1- Caraco Pharmaceuticals in Detroit, Michigan

OBSERVATION 1— *There is a failure to thoroughly review any unexplained discrepancy and the failure of a batch or any of its components to meet any of its specifications whether or not the batch has been already distributed.*

FDA expects that if there is any kind of failure investigation, that the investigation be extended to other batches, whether or not they have already been shipped. This is a very common observation across the drug industry that illustrates the lack of thorough investigations.

Reader Question:	Do you think that if a batch of drug product fails for whatever reason, one can assume that the cause of the failure cannot impact other batches? Wouldn't you want the drug company to make sure that other batches are safe to use and have the proper dosage strength and purity?

OBSERVATION 2— *There are no written procedures for production and process controls designed to assure that the drug products have the identity, strength,*

quality, and purity they purport or are represented to possess.

As stated earlier there has to be a written procedure for everything that is done and those procedures must be followed as written.

Reader Question:	Would you feel comfortable buying a drug product if the manufacturer lacked written procedures for how to make that drug or how to test it to make sure that it was the right product with the right strength? Do you think companies should have written procedures, or is it OK for firms to depend on memory or word of mouth to carry out manufacturing steps?

OBSERVATION 3— *Component weighing, measuring, and subdividing operations are not adequately supervised.*

It is expected that all steps of drug manufacturing be supervised and verified by a second person who is not the one performing the steps. This includes dispensing and weighing of active and inactive ingredients, actual manufacture of the drug product plus packaging, labeling, testing and release for shipment to commerce.

Reader Question:	How would you feel about purchasing a drug product, knowing that the manufacturer may not have added the proper ingredients or the proper amount of ingredients?

OBSERVATION 4— Batch *production and control records do not include complete information relating to the production and control of each batch.*

All steps of each operation must be documented. From an FDA standpoint, "if you didn't write it down, you didn't do it" Thorough records ensure that there is good traceability though all steps of the drug manufacturing process, which is crucial when investigating manufacturing deviations, laboratory test failure or complaints.

Reader Question:	Wouldn't it be nice to know that the drugs you are buying are manufactured using proper documentation and record keeping?

OBSERVATION 5— *Equipment and utensils are not cleaned and maintained at appropriate intervals to prevent malfunctions and contamination that would alter the safety, identity, strength, quality or purity of the drug product.*

OBSERVATION 6— *Procedures for the cleaning and maintenance of equipment are deficient regarding sufficient detail of the methods, equipment, and materials used in the cleaning and maintenance operation, and the methods of disassembly and reassembling equipment as necessary to assure proper cleaning and maintenance*

Firms are expected to have written, validated cleaning procedures for equipment and utensils that come in contact with drug product.

Reader Question:	Isn't it nice to know that the medicines you are buying may have been made using dirty equipment?

OBSERVATION 7— *Written production and process control procedures are not documented at the time of performance.*

This one warrants discussion. It is not unusual for one to perform a task and write it down later. For example, a chemist writes all his or her data on a scrap of paper and transcribes it later into their notebook after all the work has been completed, or a production operator performs several manufacturing steps and fills out the paperwork later. This kind of practice is absolutely forbidden. It could lead to mistakes, or committing fraud by changing data before recording it in an official notebook or batch record. There is a very strict requirement that all data must be recorded in an official record (laboratory notebook, manufacturing or packaging record for example) at the time it is done.

Reader Question:	Do you want to buy a drug, whose manufacturing or testing data could be fraudulent or fabricated?

OBSERVATION 8— *Employees engaged in the manufacture and processing of a drug product lack the training required to perform their assigned functions.*

OBSERVATION 9— *GMP training is not conducted on a continuing basis and with sufficient frequency to assure that employees remain familiar with CGMP requirements applicable to them.*

Reader Question:	Isn't it reassuring to know that the drugs you may have purchased were manufactured and/or tested by drug company employees who lack proper job training?

OBSERVATION 10— *Procedures describing the warehousing of drug products are not established.*

Drug products and raw materials such as active ingredients must be stored in temperature and humidity controlled conditions that will prevent deterioration or stability problems.

Major generic drug company #2- KV Pharmaceuticals in St. Louis, Missouri

Let's refer to this company as "Clueless Pharmaceuticals" and judging from the FDA 483 inspectional observations, it would appear that they are truly clueless, doing more things wrong than right. Please note that many of the observations are similar to those of Caraco Pharmaceuticals (Generic Company #1). They are also the same as observations given to just about every drug company on the planet, the difference being that most companies only get a few observations that aren't in themselves show-stoppers, whereas our friend KV Pharmaceuticals is arguably the gold standard (or maybe the lead standard) for pharmaceutical manufacturing violations.

All the observations will be listed first followed by one reader question. The actual company involved here has since been shut down for serious GMP violations,

OBSERVATION 1— *The responsibilities and procedures applicable to the quality control unit are not fully followed.*

OBSERVATION 2— *Control procedures are not established which validate the performance of those manufacturing processes that may be responsible for causing variability in the characteristics of in-process material and the drug product.*

OBSERVATION 3— *Written records are not always made of investigations into unexplained discrepancies and the failure of a batch or any of its components to meet specifications.*

OBSERVATION 4— *Written records of investigations into unexplained discrepancies and the failure of a batch or any of its components to meet specifications do not always include the conclusions and follow-up.*

OBSERVATION 5— *Investigations of an unexplained discrepancy and a failure of a batch or any of its components to meet any of its specifications did not extend to other batches of the same drug product and other drug products that may have been associated with the specific failure or discrepancy.*

OBSERVATION 6— *There is a failure to thoroughly Review any unexplained discrepancy and the failure of a batch or any of its components to meet any of its specifications whether or not the batch has been already distributed.*

OBSERVATION 7— *An NDA-Field Alert Report was not submitted within three working days of receipt of information concerning a failure of one or more distributed batches of a drug to meet the specifications established for it in the application.*

OBSERVATION 8— *An annual report did not include a full description of the manufacturing and control changes not requiring a supplemental application, listed by date in the order in which they were implemented. In an Annual Report, there is no explanation or justification for changing time release.*

OBSERVATION 9— *Drug product production and control records, are not reviewed and approved by the quality control unit to determine compliance with all established, approved written procedures before a batch is released or distributed.*

OBSERVATION 10— *Rejected closures are not controlled under a quarantine system designed to prevent their use in manufacturing or processing operations for which they are unsuitable.*

OBSERVATION 11— *Procedures describing the handling of all written and oral complaints regarding a drug product are not followed.*

OBSERVATION 12— *Changes to written procedures are not reviewed and approved by the quality control unit.*

OBSERVATION 13— *Inspection of the packaging facilities immediately before use is not done to assure that all drug products have been removed from previous operations. Specifically, line clearance practices.*

OBSERVATION 14— *Examination of packaging and labeling materials for suitability and correctness before packaging operations is not performed.*

OBSERVATION 15— *Equipment and utensils are not cleaned, maintained, and sanitized at appropriate intervals to prevent contamination that would alter the safety, identity, strength, quality or purity of the drug product.*

OBSERVATION 16— *Routine calibration of automatic, mechanical. and electronic equipment is not performed according to a written program designed to assure proper performance.*

OBSERVATION 17— *Records are not kept for the cleaning and inspection of equipment.*

OBSERVATION 18— *Procedures for the cleaning and maintenance of equipment are deficient regarding sufficient detail of the methods, equipment, and materials used in the cleaning and maintenance operation, and the methods of disassembly and reassembling equipment as necessary to assure proper cleaning and maintenance.*

OBSERVATION 19— *Written records of major equipment cleaning, maintenance, and use are not included in individual equipment logs.*

OBSERVATION 20— *Written procedures are not established and followed for the cleaning and maintenance of equipment, including utensils, used in the manufacture, processing, packing or holding of a drug product.*

OBSERVATION 21— *The building lacks adequate space for the orderly placement of equipment and materials to prevent mix-ups between different components, in-process materials, and drug products and to prevent contamination.*

OBSERVATION 22— *The written stability program does not assure testing of the drug product in*

*the same container-closure system
as that in which the drug product is
marketed.*

OBSERVATION 23— *Laboratory records do not include the
initials or signature of a second person
showing that the original records
have been reviewed for accuracy,
completeness, and compliance with
established standards.*

OBSERVATION 24— *Verification of the suitability of the
testing methods is deficient in that
they are not performed under actual
conditions of use.*

OBSERVATION 25— *Certificates of analysis from
component suppliers are accepted
in lieu of testing each component for
conformity with all appropriate written
specifications, without establishing the
reliability of the supplier's analyses
through appropriate validation of the
supplier's test results at appropriate
intervals.*

OBSERVATION 26— *Complete records are not maintained
of any modification of an established
method employed in testing.*

OBSERVATION 27— *Established laboratory control
mechanisms are not followed.*

The litany of observations is almost beyond belief. How can one company have so many problems? Cleaning is suspect, written procedures aren't followed as written, validations, i.e., assuring that a drug product can be made the same way every time so that they have consistent quality, and that test methods work the way they're supposed to, and that cleaning procedures are effective have all been called into question; plus there are potentials for mix-ups, and the quality control unit effectiveness is in question.

Reader Question:	Would you buy any drugs products that were manufactured by this company? The bad news is that this company has been in business for many years, distributing its products all over the United States. Chances are you have bought and consumed their products at one time or another. Thank your lucky stars you're still breathing.

The observations listed above are general observations from actual FDA inspection reports. For brevity, only the observations are listed. Actual inspection reports cite examples of how a violation has occurred. For example, using OBSERVATION 27 above, the observation would not just say:

"Established laboratory control mechanisms are not followed". It would be followed by the statement "For example", followed by a list of specific deficiencies.

Although this book deals mainly with generics, it is worth pointing out that generic companies are not alone in the pharmaceutical hall of shame. Brand-name companies, often referred to as "Big Pharma", sometimes have major GMP violations as well that could negatively impact your safety. One such company, McNeil Consumer Products, makes products for adults and children that are household names such as Children's Tylenol®, products that we have trusted and used for years. Let's take a look.

OBERVATION 1—   *The responsibilities and procedures applicable to the quality control unit are not fully followed.*

OBSERVATION 2—   *There are no written procedures for production   and process   controls designed to assure that the drug products have the identity, strength, quality, and purity they purport or are represented to possess.*

OBSERVATION 3— *Control procedures fail to include adequacy of mixing to assure uniformity and homogeneity.*

OBSERVATION 4— *Control procedures are not established which monitor the output and validate the performance of those manufacturing processes that may be responsible for causing variability in the characteristics of in-process material and the drug product.*

OBSERVATION 5— *Written production and process control procedures are not followed in the execution of production and process control functions.*

OBSERVATION 6— *There is a failure to thoroughly review any unexplained discrepancy whether or not the batch has been already distributed.*

OBSERVATION 7— *GMP training is not conducted with sufficient frequency to assure that employees remain familiar with CGMP requirements applicable to them.*

OBSERVATION 8— *Procedures describing the handling of all written and oral complaints regarding a drug product are not followed.*

OBSERVATION 9— *Each container of component dispensed to manufacturing is not examined by a second person to assure that the weight or measure is correct as stated in the batch records.*

OBSERVATION 10— *Strict control is not exercised over labeling issued for use in drug product labeling operations.*

OBSERVATION 11— *There is no written testing program designed to assess the stability characteristics of drug products.*

OBSERVATION 12— *Laboratory controls do not include the establishment of scientifically sound and appropriate test procedures designed to assure that components and drug products conform to appropriate standards of identity, strength, quality and purity.*

OBSERVATION 13— *Adequate lab facilities for testing and approval or rejection of components and drug products are not available to the quality control unit.*

OBSERVATION 14— *Laboratory records do not include complete records of the periodic calibration of laboratory instruments, gauges, and recording devices.*

OBSERVATION 15— *Written specifications for laboratory controls do not include a description of the sampling procedures used.*

OBSERVATION 16— *Samples taken of in-process materials for determination of conformance to specifications are not representative.*

OBSERVATION 17— *Each lot of components, was not appropriately identified as to its status in terms of being quarantined, approved or rejected.*

OBSERVATION 18— *Records are not kept for the maintenance and inspection of equipment*

OBSERVATION 19— *Strict control is not exercised over labeling issued for use in drug product labeling operations.*

OBSERVATION 20— *There is no written testing program designed to assess the stability characteristics of drug products.*

OBSERVATION 21— *Laboratory controls do not include the establishment of scientifically sound and appropriate test procedures designed to assure that components and drug products conform to appropriate standards of identity, strength, quality and purity.*

OBSERVATION 22— *Adequate lab facilities for testing and approval or rejection of components and drug products are not available to the quality control unit.*

OBSERVATION 23— *The persons double-checking the cleaning and maintenance are not dating and signing or initialing the equipment cleaning and use logs.*

OBSERVATION 24— *Records associated with drug product production and control and within the retention period for such records, were not made readily available for authorized inspection.*

OBSERVATION 25— *Written records of investigations into unexplained discrepancies do not always include the conclusions and follow-up.*

OBSERVATION 26— *Procedures describing the handling of written and oral complaints related to drug products are deficiently written or followed.*

OBSERVATION 27— *Written procedures for cleaning and maintenance fail to include description in sufficient detail of methods, equipment and materials used, description in sufficient detail of the methods of disassembling and reassembling equipment as necessary to assure proper cleaning and maintenance, and parameters relevant to the operation.*

OBSERVATION 28— *Laboratory controls do not include the establishment of scientifically sound and appropriate test procedures designed to assure that drug products conform to appropriate standards of identity, strength, quality and purity.*

OBSERVATION 29— Deviations from written test procedures are not justified.

OBSERVATION 30— *Laboratory records do not include complete records of any testing and standardization of laboratory reference standards and reagents.*

OBSERVATION 31— *Samples taken of drug products for determination of conformance to written specifications are not properly identified.*

OBSERVATION 32— *Routine inspection of mechanical and electronic equipment is not performed according to a written program designed to assure proper performance.*

OBSERVATION 33— *Written procedures are not followed for the cleaning and maintenance of equipment, including utensils, used in the manufacture, processing, packing or holding of a drug product.*

Holy cow; that's a lot of inspectional observations for a brand-name company that has been in business for years, and from whom we have been buying drug products for ourselves and for our families. These observations are clearly indicative of a company that appears to be totally out of control in terms of GMP compliance. Not good, is it?

Deficiencies included not following written procedures, not exercising appropriate responsibilities, lack of or inadequate written procedures, unsatisfactory investigation of deviations and failures, failure to meet training requirements, problems with dispensing and label control, deficient stability program (designed to assure shelf-life), deficient laboratory controls and documentation, poor control of material status identification, poor record keeping, inadequate laboratory facilities, inadequate complaint handling, problems with test procedures and records thereof. Almost every system is involved, further demonstrating systemic GMP problems. This can only result from poor quality coupled with a possible lack of commitment by upper management to both quality and compliance.

McNeil was not only issued an FDA Warning Letter, they also had to initiate a recall of many of its products.

WARNING LETTERS:

As previously mentioned, if a drug company gets through an FDA inspection with no 483 or a light 483 with only a few observations, FDA will allow voluntary corrections of deficiencies, and will verify those corrections during their next inspection.

On the other hand, if an inspection reveals serious deficiencies that could affect or even just potentially affect consumer safety, FDA may issue a Warning Letter to the firm. Once again, Warning Letters are no fun and should be avoided if possible. They impact a firm's reputation and can affect its ability to get government contracts or new drug application approvals. They can also eventually lead to recalls or more severe regulatory action by FDA.

Warning Letters are public record and are posted on FDA's website at www.fda.gov. New warning letters are posted every Tuesday. Warning letters going back years are available for viewing any time. They can be searched a number of ways such as by most recent, by year or by company. It's real easy to see who's been naughty and who's been nice. Chapter 6, "Self Defense", will show you how to use the FDA website to investigate companies before buying their products; not only for drugs, but for foods, medical devices and biologics (blood products).

Now it's time to name some more names. The following Table, covering a period of time up to this writing shows company name, date issued and reason for getting the warning letter. The Table is sorted by most recent first. Make note of the company names listed in Table 1, some may surprise you.

Table 1

Letter Issue Date	Company Name	Reason
August 03, 2010	Cosmed Labs, Inc.	CGMP for Finished Pharmaceuticals/Adulterated/Misbranded
July26, 2010	Nitrox Inc.	CGMP for Finished Pharmaceuticals/Adulterated/Misbranded
July 20, 2010	Haw Par Healthcare, Ltd.	CGMP for Finished Pharmaceuticals/OTC Drug Manufacturing/Adulterated/Misbranded
June 29, 2010	Hi-Tech Pharmacal Co., Inc.	CGMP for Finished Pharmaceuticals/Adulterated/Misbranded
June 21, 2010	Corepharma,LLC.	Current Good Manufacturing Practice Regulation for Finished Pharmaceuticals
June 18, 2010	BENEV	Current Good Manufacturing Practice Regulation for Finished Pharmaceuticals/Adulterated
May 27, 2010	Ribbon SRL	CGMP Regulation for Finished Pharmaceuticals/Adulterated

Letter Issue Date	Company Name	Reason
May 21, 2010	AVEVA Drug Delivery Systems, Inc.	CGMP Regulation for Finished Pharmaceuticals/ Adulterated
May 21, 2010	K.C. Pharmaceuticals, Inc.	CGMP/QSR/Medical Devices/Finished Pharmaceuticals/Adulterated
May 20, 2010	River's Edge Pharmaceuticals LLC	CGMP for Finished Pharmaceuticals/Adulterated/ Misbranded
May 10, 2010	Braintree Laboratories, Inc.	CGMP For Manufacturing, Processing, Packing, Storage & Holding/Adulterated
April 12, 2010	Hospira, Inc.	CGMP for Finished Pharmaceuticals/Deviations/ Adulterated
April 03, 2010	Shamrock Medical Solutions, Inc.,.	CGMP for Finished Pharmaceuticals/Misbranded/ Adulterated
March 30, 2010	Coates International Holdings, Inc.	CGMP Manufacture, Processing, Packing or Holding/Adulterated

Letter Issue Date	Company Name	Reason
March 29, 2010	Apotex, Inc.	CGMP for Finished Pharmaceuticals/Adulterated
March 26, 2010	Pierre Fabre Medicament Production	CGMP for Finished Pharmaceuticals/Adulterated
March 10, 2010	ISTA Pharmaceuticals, Inc.	Labeling/Promotional Claims False & Misleading/ Misbranded
Feb 23, 2010	Tri-Med Laboratories, Inc,	Current Good Manufacturing Practice Regulation for Finished Pharmaceuticals
Feb 18, 2010	Vertical Pharmaceuticals	Premarket Approval/Misbranded/Adulterated
Feb 17, 2010	Unisource, Inc.	Unapproved New Drug/Misbranded
Feb 8, 2010	Poly Pharmaceuticals, Inc.	New Drug/Adulterated

Letter Issue Date	Company Name	Reason
Feb 8, 2010	Jaymac Pharmaceuticals LLC	New Drug/Adulterated
Feb 8, 2010	Edwards Pharmaceutical, Inc.	New Drug/Adulterated New Drug/Adulterated
Feb 8, 2010	Magna Pharmaceuticals, Inc.	Labeling/False & Misleading Claims/New Drug/ Misbranded
Feb 5, 2010	Lily del Caribe, Inc	CGMP/Active Pharmaceutical Ingredients/ Adulterated
Feb 4, 2010	Kirk Pharmaceuticals LLC	CGMP for Finished Pharmaceuticals/Adulterated
Feb 2, 2010	Portal Pharmaceutical,Inc.	Labeling/New Drug Application
Jan 28,. 2010	Xian Libang Pharmaceutical Co., Ltd.	CGMP/Manufacturing Facility/Active Pharmaceutical Ingredient

Letter Issue Date	Company Name	Reason
Jan 15, 2010	McNeil Specialty and Consumer Pharmaceuticals	CGMP Regulations for Finished Pharmaceuticals/ Adulterated
Jan 15, 2010	Baxter Biosciences	CGMP Deviations
Jan 14, 2010	Sunrise Pharmaceutical, Inc.	CGMP for Finished Pharmaceuticals/Adulterated/ Misbranded
Dec 22, 2009	Balchem Corporation	Current Good Manufacturing Practice Regulation for Finished Pharmaceuticals
Dec 21, 2010	Ohm Laboratories, Inc.	CGMP for Finished Pharmaceuticals/Adulterated
Dec 11, 2009	Teva Parenterals Medicines, Inc.	CGMP for Finished Pharmaceuticals/Adulterated
Dec 9, 2009	M W Laboratories, Inc,	OTC Drug Labeling/New Drug/Misbranded

Letter Issue Date	Company Name	Reason
Nov 30, 2009	Aluwe, LLC	Unapproved New Drug/Misbranded
Nov 27, 2009	GDMI, Inc	CGMP for Finished Pharmaceuticals/Adulterated/Misbranded
Nov 20, 2009	Wellspring International, Inc.	Unapproved New Drug
Nov 13, 2009	Cornerstone Therapeutics, Inc.	Labeling/Promotional Claims False & Misleading/Misbranded
Ditto	Allegis Pharmaceuticals LLC	Lacks Approved New Drug Application/Adulterated
Ditto	Tiber Laboratories	Lacks Approved New Drug Application/Adulterated
Ditto	Everett Laboratories	Lacks Approved New Drug Application/Adulterated

Letter Issue Date	Company Name	Reason
Ditto	Larken Laboratories	Lacks Approved New Drug Application/Adulterated
Ditto	Victory Pharma, Inc.	Lacks Approved New Drug Application/Adulterated
Ditto	Zyber Pharmaceuticals, Inc.	Lacks Approved New Drug Application/Adulterated
Ditto	Accentia Biopharmaceuticals, Inc.	Lacks Approved New Drug Application/Adulterated
Ditto	Wraser Pharmaceuticals	Lacks Approved New Drug Application/Adulterated
Nov 9, 2009	Providence Pharmaceuticals LLC	CGMP for Finished Pharmaceuticals/Misbranded/Adulterated
Oct 23, 2009	ZaCH Systems S.A.	CGMP Manufacture, Processing, Packing or Holding/Adulterated
Sept 28, 2009	Drugs Are Us, Inc.	Active Pharmaceutical Ingredient/Adulterated

The Warning Letter list given in Table 1 serves to point out that there are common themes from company to company such as GMP violations, labeling problems and distributing unapproved drugs.

GMP violations are widespread among many firms. Not all companies that receive 483s get Warning Letter because their violations are not significant enough to be a threat to consumer safety. If one reads various 483s and Warning Letters, it becomes quite evident that everyone seems to get cited for the same stuff. So similar are Warning Letters, that one could pretty much interchange company names on a typical Warning Letter and it would read the same. Table 2 and Figure 1 illustrate the distribution of Warning Letters listed in Table 1 by category and by type of company.

Table 2

WARNING LETTERS – PERCENTAGE BY TYPE	
Reason	Percentage
GMP Violations	59.6
Unapproved New Drug	23.4
Misbranded-Adulterated	10.6
Labeling	6.5

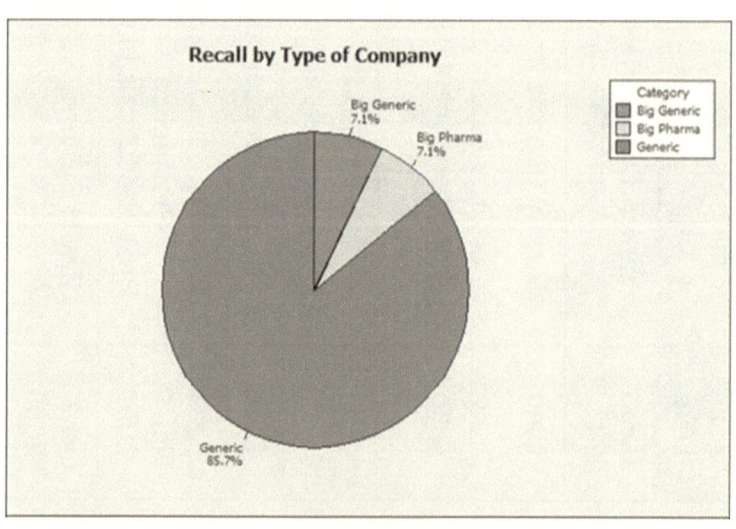

Figure 1

Table 2 clearly indicates that most of the Warning Letters for the period represented are a result of GMP violations. Looking at the distribution for the same period by type of company (Figure 1), it is clear that most of the Warning Letters were issued to generic companies. Remember these facts when reading Chapter 3, "Drug Approvals and the Generic World".

GMP problems are prevalent among Warning Letter recipients. The following section from an actual Warning Letter helps make the point:

1. *Your firm has not thoroughly investigated any unexplained discrepancy or the failure of a batch or any of its components to meet its specifications whether or not the batch has already been distributed [21 C.F.R. § 211.192]. For example,*

    a. *Your quality control unit (QCD) has not conducted out-of-specification (OOS) investigations for products that failed to meet bulk drug specifications (e.g., appearance, pH, and microbial contamination). Specifically, your QCD did not conduct OOS investigations for the OOS bulk drug TD+S Sunscreen. However, you used this inprocess bulk drug product to manufacture TD+S Sunscreen **(b)(4)**. Further, this product was released and distributed.*

    b. *In your December 31, 2009 response, you provided a revised Standard Operating Procedure (SOP) #**(b)(4)**, "Out Of Specification (OOS) Procedure." Your response is inadequate because the SOP does not describe the steps that will be taken to investigate OOS results (e.g., laboratory testing procedures, production process review).*

    This is a repeat violation from the inspection conducted in 2006.

    c. *Your QCD reviewed and approved the distribution of a drug product that was manufactured using expired components. You fulfilled an order request from your customer by altering the lot number for expired Salicylic Acid Exfoliator 30%. Although a deviation investigation was conducted, the investigation was not thorough (e.g., identification of other affected lots, root cause determination, and corrective and preventive actions).*

43

In your December 31, 2009, and February 8, 2010 responses, you state that you have "adjusted the system so that there are inventory controls that must be adhered to that have fail-safe controls built in" (sic). Your response is inadequate because you have neither described the inventory controls nor have you provided any documents to demonstrate that these changes have occurred (e.g., SOPs). In addition, you have not provided any information regarding the investigation of the incident. Although you state that the discrepancy was a "one-time incident," you have not indicated how your firm has reached this conclusion. In addition, you have not addressed the QCD's inadequate review of drug product production and controls. Further, you have not indicated whether you performed a review of other products that may have also been affected.

2. *Your film failed to follow procedures for the handling of all written and oral complaints regarding a drug product, including specific complaint information or a reason that an investigation was found not to be necessary. [21 C.F.R. § 211.198]. For example,*

   a. *You failed to ensure that the Complaint Review Form, required by SOP#(b)(4), "Complaint Handling," was used to document complaints. Significantly, your complaint records lacked: (1) product name; (2) lot number; (3) date of the event; (4) results of investigations; and (5) an evaluation of the seriousness of the complaint.*

      In your December 31, 2009, and February 8, 2010 responses, you state that you have created a new complaint investigation form (Form (b)(4) "Complaint Investigation") and have trained personnel regarding its use. However, your response is inadequate because the revised SOP# (b)(4) and/or the new form do not include provisions for review to determine whether a complaint represents a serious and unexpected adverse drug experience subject to the reporting requirements under 21 C.F.R. §§ 310.305 and 514.80.

      This is a repeat violation from the inspection conducted in 2006.

b. *You failed to document the reasons that investigations were not necessary for product complaints attributed to adverse reactions or product quality issues as recorded in your complaint log and product return list.*

Your revised SOP#(b)(4), "Complaint Handling," states that the complaint information will be investigated and reviewed by your QCU upon receipt. Your revised SOP is inadequate because you do not require the documentation of a reason that an investigation was found unnecessary or the name of the responsible person making that determination.

3. *Your firm failed to reject any lot of components that did not meet the appropriate written specifications for identity, strength, quality and purity [21 C.F.R. § 211.84(e)].*

For example, a benzoyl peroxide raw material (lot (b)(4)) failed to meet specifications and was not rejected. The raw material was subsequently used to manufacture Acne Spot Treatment (b)(4)). These lots were released and distributed.

In your December 31, 2009, and February 8, 2010 responses, you state that this was a "one time incident." Your response is inadequate because you have not indicated how this conclusion was made or provided any information regarding the investigation of the incident.

4. *Your firm does not have adequate written procedures for production and process controls designed to assure that the drug products you manufacture have the identity, strength, quality, and purity they purport or are represented to possess [21 C.F.R. § 211.100(a)]. For example, you have not validated the manufacturing processes for the following drug products: Salicylic Acid Exfoliator 30%; Numbscents Topical Analgesic Butter (lidocaine HCl, benzocaine); Polyclear Tretinoin Cream; Skin Smoothing Moisturizer (hydroquinone); Salicylic Cleanser; Pure Titanium Dioxide (sunscreen); and Acne Spot Treatment (benzoyl peroxide). Further, your validation studies titled "Hydroquinone Skin Lightening Formula (Protocol (b)(4)," and "TD+S Sunscreen SPF-30 (Protocol (b)(4)," are inadequate because they do not include raw data,1 and an adequate evaluation of critical quality attributes.*

Your December 31, 2009, and February 8, 2010 responses are inadequate because they fail to address process validation for the listed drug products.

This is a repeat violation from the inspection conducted in 2006.

5. *Your firm failed to prepare batch production and control records for each batch of drug product produced that includes an accurate reproduction of the appropriate master production or control record [21 C.F.R. § 211.188(a)] and documentation of weights and measures of components used in the course of processing to demonstrate that each significant step in the manufacture and processing of the batch was accomplished [21 C.F.R. § 211.188(b)(4)]. For example,*

   a. *Your TD+S Sunscreen SPF-30 specifications for* **(b)(4)** *listed in the batch record are inconsistent with the specifications in the master batch record. Your QCD could not provide a justification for these inconsistencies.*

   In your December 31, 2009, and February 8, 2010 responses, you indicate that batch records have been updated to ensure that they contain all necessary specifications. You also state that you will assess the appropriateness of specifications. However, you have not indicated that you will perform a global review of all drug products to ensure that master production and control records include complete manufacturing and control instructions.

   b. *Your control and batch records (and master production records) do not include the weights or measures of active ingredients and raw materials used in the manufacture of your drug products (e.g., Nutracine Tinted Sunscreen SPF 30 and Skin Smoothing Moisturizer (Hydroquinone)).*

   We acknowledge your response dated December 31, 2009, wherein you state that you have added an **(b)(4)**, *column on all manufacturing batch records. Your response is not adequate because the master production and control and batch records with* **(b)(4)**, *columns were not available during the follow-up inspection dated January 2 - 4, 2010, and were not provided in your February 8, 2010 response.*

6. *Your film does not have an adequate written testing program designed to assess the stability characteristics of drug products in order to determine appropriate storage conditions and expiration dates [21 C.F.R. § 211.166(a)]. For example,*

   a. *The analytical methods used in your stability studies are not stability-indicating. Your SOP# **(b)(4)** "Stability Testing," fails to require analyses that (1) identify degradation products or (2) demonstrate the effect of temperature, humidity, oxidation, and light on the drug products.*

   *Your firm established expiration dates for drug products without a scientific rationale. Your real-time stability data for Face Sunblock SPF-25 revealed that 2 out of 3 stability lots **(b)(4)** did not meet the specification for assay at the 12-month test point. You did not investigate the stability failure. However, your firm approved the product expiration for 1 year. In addition, your firm failed to retain sufficient stability samples to conduct a complete analysis for Face Sunblock SPF-25 **(b)(4)***

   Your December 31, 2009, and February 8, 2010 responses are inadequate because you have not specified the stability-indicating tests that will be performed. Although a revised stability testing SOP was provided, you have not provided evidence of stability chamber validation. Further, as a corrective action, you changed the "shelf life" of SPF-25; however, you did not provide stability testing data to support this change. Stability testing of all marketed lots should be performed to assure that the distributed products have the appropriate expiration dates.

   This is a repeat violation from the inspection conducted in 2006.

7. *Your firm has not conducted at least one specific identity test and has not established the reliability of the supplier's analyses through appropriate validation of the supplier's test results at appropriate intervals [21 C.F.R. § 211.84(d)(2)].*

   For example, you accepted reports of analysis from suppliers for components labeled as "Lidocaine USP," "Tretinoin USP," "Titanium Dioxide USP," and "Benzoyl Peroxide USP," without conducting at least one specific identity test. In addition, you have not provided documentation demonstrating that you have established the reliability of the supplier's analysis through appropriate validation of the supplier's test results at appropriate intervals.

Your December 31, 2009, and February 8, 2010 responses are inadequate because you have not explained how you will assess the reliability of your supplier's analysis.

This is a repeat observation from the inspection conducted in 2006.

8. *Your film has not established written procedures for cleaning and maintenance of equipment [21 C.F.R. § 211.67(b)].*

   Your cleaning validation was limited to the cleaning process of a plastic 55-gallon drum used in the manufacture of Hydroquinone Skin Lightening Formula. You have not established an adequate rationale, including determining whether this product is the most difficult product to clean. The validation also does not include other equipment used in the manufacture and packing of this product.

   We acknowledge your December 31, 2009 response that describes your cleaning validation protocols and that cleaning validation will be performed on all equipment used to manufacture OTC products. However, during the follow-up inspection dated January 2 - 4, 2010, your cleaning validation protocols were not available. Further, your February 8, 2010 response provided an incomplete cleaning validation protocol for one piece of equipment. In addition, it was not clear whether cleaning validation will still be performed on other equipment.

   This is a repeat observation from the inspection conducted in 2006.

9. *You failed to ensure that each person engaged in the manufacture, processing, packing, or holding of a drug product has the education, training, and experience, or any combination thereof, to enable that person to perform their assigned functions [21 C.F.R. § 211.25(a)].*

   For example, your "QC/ R&D Chemist" has not been trained to perform specific tasks such as microbial limits testing under USP <61>.

   We acknowledge your December 31, 2009, and February 8, 2010 responses, wherein you state that you will conduct CGMP and SOP staff training biannually with "real time" updates. During the January 2 - 4, 2010 follow-up inspection, we observed that you have begun training production and laboratory personnel. Your response is inadequate because you have not established completion dates and training programs for current good manufacturing practices and SOPs. In addition, your statement regarding "real time" update training remains unclear.

This is a repeat violation from the inspection conducted in 2006.

Yes, this is typical stuff that you'll see over and over again on FDA Warning Letters. It seems that many companies have gone to the same school to learn how not to do things right. Let's look at one more example. Looks like "same song, different arrangement".

Specific violations observed during the inspection include, but are not limited to, the following:

1. *Your firm does not have, for each batch of drug product, appropriate laboratory determination of satisfactory conformance to final specifications for the drug product, including the identity and strength of each active ingredient, prior to release [21 C.F.R. § 211.165(a)]. For example, your firm does not perform finished product testing on filled cylinders of Dolonox, a 50% USP Nitrous Oxide and 50% USP Oxygen compressed medical gas mixture, prior to release. From September 2003 to May 2009, your firm released* **(b)(4)** *high-pressure cylinders of Dolonox without testing the product for identity and strength.*

2. *Your firm has not established scientifically sound and appropriate specifications, standards, sampling plans, and test procedures designed to assure that drug products conform to appropriate standards of identity, strength, quality, and purity [21 C.F.R. § 211.160(b)].*

    For example, your firm has not established appropriate written procedures to test liquid Nitrogen NF for assay and limit of Oxygen. Your firm's only written Standard Operating Procedure (SOP) for testing liquid Nitrogen NF specifies that the Splitter Test is to be used for identity testing. The Splitter Test is not considered a scientifically sound test method. Further, during the inspection, you *told our investigators that the standard practice for assay testing of liquid Nitrogen NF was to use **(b)(4)** handheld analyzers. However, you could not provide documentation of **(b)(4)** handheld analyzer testing. Please note that the FDA does not consider the **(b)(4)** handheld analyzer to be an acceptable test method for the assay of liquid Nitrogen NF because your firm has not demonstrated that it is equivalent to the monograph test method for assay.*

3. *Your firm did not prepare batch production and control records for each batch of drug product produced, including documentation that each significant step in the manufacture, processing, packing, or holding of the batch was accomplished [21 C.F.R. § 211.188(b)]. For example, your firm manufactures Dolonox without producing batch production and control records to document performance of the necessary cylinder prefill checks such as visual examination, dead ring test for corrosion, prefill odor check, and vacuum evacuation.*

4. *Your firm does not have adequate written procedures for production and process controls designed to assure that the drug products you manufacture have the identity, strength, quality, and/or purity they purport or are represented to possess [21 C.F.R. § 211.100(a)]. For example, your firm has not established written procedures for the manufacturing, testing, and distribution of Dolonox.*

5. *Your firm did not have drug product production and control records reviewed and approved by a Quality Control Unit (QCD) to determine compliance with all established, approved written procedures before a batch is released or distributed [21 C.F.R. § 211.192]. For example, your firm's QCU did not review or approve batch production records for liquid Nitrogen NF distributed between November 24, 2009, and February 19, 2010.*

6. *Your firm did not follow written production and process control procedures in the execution of the various production and process control functions [21 C.F.R. § 211.100(b)]. For example, SOP "Medical Gas Supplier Audit Report" requires your Firm to audit your medical gas supplier every However, your firm has not conducted audits of your supplier of liquid Nitrogen NF.*

Nothing has changed over the years with regards to Warning Letter content. Companies that are screw-ups, are simply screw-ups and that's all there is to it. The companies in Table 1 are drug companies, most of whom you probably never heard of. These companies that you haven't heard of, could be making active ingredients that go into drug products you buy, or they could be contract manufacturers who supply drug products to drug chains or discount stores. Isn't that just great? We don't know for sure if the company who made the drugs we buy has gotten a Warning Letter or recall notice.

Table 1 only deals with drug company Warning Letters over a 12-month period, but during that period, a plethora of Warning Letters were also issued to food companies and medical device companies for violations of standards governing those industries. As a matter of fact, in the first six months of 2010 alone, FDA issued over 300 Warning Letters, in 2009, over 550.

OK, we have looked at 483s (inspection reports) and Warning Letters. Now let's explore the ugly world of product recalls. All kinds of products are recalled every week. This includes cosmetics, foods, drugs, medical devices, biologics (blood products) and veterinary products. Recalls are actually scarier than Warning Letters, because it means that something that has a problem is already on the market and that we could have used that product, perhaps resulting in serious consequences.

There are a number of reasons for recalls such as not manufacturing according to GMPs, shelf-life problems, mislabeling, mix-ups, sub potent of super potent (too little or too much active ingredient), or chemical, foreign material or microbiological contamination. Recalls are categorized according to degree of seriousness with a Class I recall being the most serious, and a Class 3 the least serious. A Class 1 is assigned when use of the product could have serious consequences including hospitalization or even death. Enforcement reports listing all recalls are published on FDA's website every Wednesday. It makes for interesting reading and can give you, the consumer, a tip-off as to what not to buy at your local supermarket or pharmacy. It is also useful for checking your household drug inventory to see is you have any recalled products lying around.

Table 3 lists a number of drug recalls, citing company name and class of recall and reason. The actual items recalled are too numerous to list. I will leave it up to you, the reader, to check out FDA's website. More on this in Chapter 6, "Self Defense".

Table 3

Manufacturing Company	Class	Reason
Atlas Operations ,Inc.	1	Unapproved Drug Application
Perrigo Florida, Inc.	2	Label Mix-up
Teva	2	Product may exhibit discoloration
Caraco	2	Impurities/Degradation products
McNeil Consumer Health Care	2	Chemical Contamination
Proctor and Gamble	2	Precipitate in product
Allergan	3	Failed pH specification
Novapharm	2	Subpotent
Jayhawk Pharmacy & Patient Supply	2	Lack of conformance with cGMPs
Biovail Corp.	3	Extended release failed release rate.
G&W Laboratories	3	Stability failure
Apotex, Inc.	2	Active ingredient used that had a failing impurity level.
Gasco Industrial	2	Lack of cGMPS
Paddock Labs	2	Stability failure at 12 months
McNeil Healthcare	2	Failed dissolution
Vintage Pharmaceuticals	2	Sub-potent
F&F Foods	3	Sub-potent
Mallinckrodt	3	cGMP Deviations

Manufacturing Company	Class	Reason
Pfizer	3	Impurities/Degradation products
Claris Lifesciences Ltd	1	Non-Sterility
Patheon Puerto Rico, Inc.	2	Chemical Contamination
Claris Lifesciences Ltd	1	Non-Sterility
Schawrz Pharma Manufacturing, Inc.	2	Tablet Thickness; presence of thicker, overweight tablets due to presence of start-up waste in acceptable product.
West-ward Pharmaceutical	3	Dissolution failure
Matrix Initiatives	1	Adverse event, loss of smell.
McNeil Consumer Healthcare	2	cGMP Deficiencies
Aurobindo	2	Adulterated by Presence of foreign tablets
Aurobindo	2	Tablets too thick
Altaire Pharmaceuticals	3	Defective container
McNeil Consumer Healthcare	2	Chemical contamination
Nitrox	2	Marketed without approved drug application
Glenmark Generics Ltd.	3	Incorrect or missing package insert
DSM Pharmaceuticals	2	Impurities/Degradation products
McNeil Consumer Healthcare	2	Labeling, incorrect, missing lot number
Hospira, Inc.	1	Presence of particulate matter
AnazaoHealth Corp	1	Adverse event, such as lid swelling, periorbital cellulitis and chemosis.

Manufacturing Company	Class	Reason
Luitpold Pharmaceuticals	1	Presence of particulate matter
Rentschler Biotechnologie Gmbh & Co. KG	2	Lack of assurance of sterility
Corepharma LLC	2	Tablets have the potential to contain metal particulates
McNeil Consumer Healthcare	2	Chemical Contamination
Actavis Mid Atlantic LLC	2	Impurities/Degradation Products: Out-of-specification (OOS) stability results for hydrocortisone related compounds.
Teva Animal Health	2	cGMP violations
Teva Parenteral Medicines	2	Impurities/Degradation products
Nycomed USA Inc.	2	Potential bacterial contamination
Apotex Corp	2	Failed pH specification
McNeil Consumer Healthcare	2	Chemical contamination
Special Care Home Oxygen & Medical Equipment, Inc	2	cGMP Deviations
Mallinckrodt	2	Lack of efficacy
Hickma Farmaceutica	2	Lack of stability
H2O Plus LP	3	Error with regard to preservative
Nanjing Pharmaceutical Factory Co., Ltd	2	cGMP Deviations
Ben-Venue Laboratories	2	Lack of Sterility
Cadista Pharmaceuticals, Inc.	2	Stability failure
Rugby Laboratories	2	Miscalibrated and/or defective delivery system
Amneal Pharmaceuticals	2	Subpotent

Manufacturing Company	Class	Reason
LNK International, Inc.	2	Mislabeleing
Barr Labs	2	Some capsules do not meet dissolution specifications
Haloteco	1	Marketed without an approved drug application
Proctor & Gamble	1	Microbial contamination of non-sterile product
Accucaps Industries LTD	2	Labeling mix-up
Kirk Pharmaceuticals	2	Kirk Pharmaceuticals is recalling Diphenhydramine Hydrochloride 25mg capsules, for sub-potent assay results due to improper storage conditions of the product during transit.
Schering-Plough	2	Impurities/Degradation products
Abbott Laboratories	2	Unit dose mispacking
Noven Pharmaceuticals, Inc.	2	Miscalibrated and/or Defective Delivery System
Lannett Company	2	Failed USP dissolution test requirements
USV Limited	2	Adulterated presence of foreign tablets
Wyeth	3	Cross-contamination with other products
Pfiizer	3	Failed USP dissolution test requirements
AVEVA Drug Delivery Systems	3	Impurities/Degradation products
APP Pharmaceuticals LLP	3	Impurities/Degradation products

Manufacturing Company	Class	Reason
Coates International Holdings	3	Product was distributed without proper stability data to support the 2 year shelf-life
Paddock Laboratories	2	Failing dissolution at 6-month
Novartis Pharmaceuticals	2	Combination capsule missing one ingredient
Kirk Pharmaceuticals	2	Kirk Pharmaceuticals is recalling Diphenhydramine Hydrochloride 25mg capsules, for sub-potent assay results due to improper storage conditions of the product during transit.
Cadista Pharmaceuticals, Inc.	3	Pharmaceutical may have been packaged with two dosage strengths of the same drug.
Coates International Holdings	3	Sample product failed 6-month ambient test points for assay of active ingredient.
HALOTECO	1	Marketed without an approved drug application
Wyeth	3	Cross-contamination with other products
Corepharma LLC	2	One lot of Pilocarpine Hydrochloride Tablets, 5 mg may contain out of specification tablets for weight and thickness.
L. Perrigo Co.	3	Misbranded
Wyeth	3	Drug does not conform to dissolution specification
Rockline Industries	3	Subpotent

Manufacturing Company	Class	Reason
Amgen Manufaturing	2	Lack of assurance of sterility
Dentsply Caulk	3	12-month stability failure
Sandoz	3	Marketed without an approved drug application
IGA, Inc.	3	Subpotent
L. Perrigo Co.	3	Misbranded
L. Perrigo Co.	2	Mislabeling
Luitpold Pharmaceuticals, Inc.	2	Out-of-specification product for aluminum levels
Gilead Sciences	2	Product stability may have been compromised due to defective refrigeration storage unit.
McNeil Consumer Healthcare	2	Chemical Contamination
L. Perrigo Co.	2	Label mix-up

Figure 2 shown below, representing the recalls listed in Table 3, once again illustrating that most of the problems lie with generic companies.

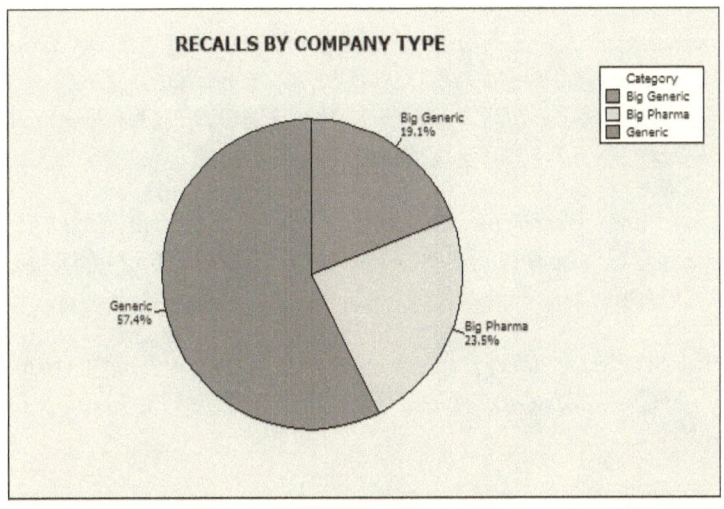

Figure 2

Remember this also when reading Chapter 3.

The recalls listed in Table 3 are all in 2010. Some are minor, while others are more serious and very widespread. Table 2 clearly shows that some companies like McNeil Consumer Healthcare have had serious problems. McNeil's recalls were widely publicized in the press and on FDA's website   Needless to say, these recalls have cost the company a lot of money, and I suspect fairly serious damage to their reputation as well. Let's look at an actual recall listing from the FDA's enforcement report of June 2, 2010.

PRODUCT

1) Concentrated Tylenol Infants' Drops, (Acetaminophen), 80 mg, a) 1/2 oz Bottle Dropper (UPC 300450122155 and UPC 350580144183), b) 1 oz Bottle Dropper (UPC 300450122018 and UPC Code 300450122100), OTC, Grape Flavor. Recall # D-550-2010;

2) Concentrated Tylenol Infants' Drops (Acetaminophen), 80 mg, 1 oz Bottle Dropper, OTC, Dye Free, Cherry Flavor, UPC 300450167118 and 300450167019. Recall # D-551-2010;

3) Concentrated Tylenol Infants' Drops(Acetaminophen), 80 mg, a)1/2 oz Bottle Dropper (UPC 300450186157); b) 1 oz Bottle Dropper (UPC 300450186300), OTC, Cherry Flavor. Recall # D-552-2010;

4) Concentrated Motrin Infants' Drops (Ibuprofen), 50 mg, a) 1/2 oz Bottle Dropper (UPC 300450198150), b) 1 oz Bottle Dropper (UPC 300450198013 and UPC 300450198112), OTC, Dye-Free, Original Berry Flavor. Recall # D-553-2010;

5) Concentrated Motrin Infants' Drops, (Ibuprofen), 50 mg, 1/2 OZ Bottle Dropper, OTC, Original Berry Flavor, UPC 300450524157. Recall # D-554-2010;

6) Children's Zyrtec Allergy, (Cetirizine HCl) Allergy, 1 mg, Syrup 1/2 oz Bottle, OTC, Bubble Gum, UPC Code 300450205155. Recall # D-555-2010;

7) Johnson's Baby Relief Kit, OTC, which contains Concentrated Tylenol Infants Drops, 1/2 oz Bottle Dropper, Grape and Concentrated Motrin

Infants Drops 1/2 oz Bottle Dropper, Berry, UPC Code 381370026426. Recall # D-556-2010

CODE

1) Lot numbers: a) AAM004, AAM021, ABM030, SDM124, SEM051, SFM027, SHM018, SJM130, SLM105, SMM059, SMM072, SMM152, and SSM040, and AAM062, SDM123, SJM131, SMM005, SPM008, SSM003, and SSM034; b) AAM099, SEM099, SFM003, SJM088, SMM009, SMM082, SSM019, SSM080; and SDM079, SDM080, SDM081, SDM100, SDM101, SEM047, SJM015, SJM089 and SJM162;

2) Lot numbers: SDM097, SDM129, SDM130, SDM131, SEM046, SHM042, SHM061, SJM057, SJM157, and SMM008; and AAM005, AAM085, AAM120, SDM128, SEM098, SFM004, SFM005, SFM006, SHM024, SHM041, SJM087, SJM189, SLM038, SLM039, SLM110, SLM111, SLM112, SMM068, SMM083, SPM038, SPM065, and SSM018;

3) Lot numbers: a) AAM093, SDM093, SEM050, SEM113, SHM032, SJM049, SLM052, SLM104, SMM043, SMM073, SPM009, SPM059, and SSM061; b) SJM137, SLM113, and SPM039;

4) Lot numbers: a) SCM079, SEM072, SJM081, SMM004, SMM166, and SSM072, b) SDM010, SDM011, SDM037, SDM132, SEM048, SEM079, SEM080, SEM101, SEM120, SEM121, SEM122, SEM123, SHM033, SJM056, SJM090, SLM058, SLM059, SLM060, SMM010, SMM011, SMM066, SMM067, SSM048, SSM067; and SDM098, SDM099, SEM049, SEM100, SFM007, SFM008, SFM009, SHM062, SJM055, and SJM158;

5) Lot numbers: AAM118, AAM119, SDM031, SDM069, SDM092, SEM071, SJM007, SLM053, SMM003, SMM044, SMM167, SSM012, and SSM062;

6) Lot numbers: SMM153, SPC019, SPC022, SPC023, SPM010, and SPM010A;

7) Lot numbers: 2058J, 2748J, 2808J, 2818J, 3088J, 3098J, 3438J, 3458J, 0129J, 0149J, 0709J, 0719J, 0729J, 0759J,

0969J, 0979J, 0989J, 2059J, 2089J, 2109J, 2119J, and 2449J

RECALLING FIRM/MANUFACTURER

McNeil Consumer Healthcare, Div of McNeil-PPC, Inc., Fort Washington, PA, by letters on March 29, 2010. Firm initiated recall is ongoing.

REASON

Labeling: Incorrect/Missing Lot No.(s): There is a potential for the product lot number and/or expiration date to become illegible on the bottle label.

VOLUME OF PRODUCT IN COMMERCE

18,707,407 bottles, droppers and 66,560 kits

DISTRIBUTION

Nationwide; Dominican Republic, Trinidad & Tobago, Guatemala, Jamaica, Maite, UAE, and Kuwait

How about recalls reported in the FDA's enforcement report of August 11, 2010.

PRODUCT

Motrin IB (Ibuprofen) Tablets USP 200 mg, 100 count bottle, OTC, NDC 50580-109-04, UPC 3 0045 0463 04 3. Recall # D-715-2010;

2) Motrin IB (Ibuprofen) Caplets, USP 200 mg, a) 24 count bottle, NDC 50580-110-03, UPC 3 0045 0481 030; b) Bonus pack (50+ 25) count bottle, NDC 50580-110-76, UPC 3 0045 0481 764; OTC. Recall # D-716-2010;

3) Benadryl (Diphenhydramine HCl) Allergy tablets, 25 mg each, 100 Ultratab bottle, OTC, NDC 50580-226-10; UPC 3 12547 17033 8. Recall # D-717-2010;

4) Tylenol (Acetaminophen) Tablets, Extra Strength, 500 mg Each, Easy to Swallow EZ Tabs, a) 50 count bottle, NDC 50580-422-50, UPC 3 00450422507; b) 225 count NDC 50580-422-37, UPC 3 00450422378, OTC. Recall # D-718-2010;

5) Children's Tylenol (Acetaminophen) Tablets, Meltaways, Bubblegum Burst flavor, 80 mg, 30 count bottle, OTC, NDC 50580-519-30, UPC

3-0045-0519-306. Recall # D-719-2010;

6) Tylenol (Acetaminophen) Caplets, Extra Strength, 500 mg each a) 24 count bottle, NDC 50580-710-24, UPC 3 0045-0444-240, b) 24+12 count bottle, NDC 50580-449-31, UPC 3 0045-0444-318, c) 50 count bottle, NDC 50580-449-06, UPC 3 0045-0444-530, d) 50 count bottle, This Package for Households Without Young Children, NDC 50580-449-07, UPC 3 0045-0449-07 8, OTC. Recall # D-720-2010;

7) Tylenol (Acetaminophen) Capsules, Extra Strength, Rapid Release, 500 mg each, a) 225 count, NDC 50580-488-25, UPC 3 0045 0488 251, b) 24 count, NDC, 50580-488-24, UPC 3 0045 0488 244), OTC. Recall # D-721-2010;

8) Tylenol PM (Acetaminophen/Diphenhydramine HCl) Caplets, Extra Strength, 500mg/25 mg, a) 24 count bottle, NDC 50580-482-24, UPC 3 0045-0482-242, b) Day & Night Value Pack, 50 count bottle, NDC 50580-527-10, UPC 3 0045-0527-103, OTC. Recall # D-722-2010;

9) Tylenol PM (Acetaminophen/Diphenhydramine HCl) Geltab, Extra Strength, 500 mg/25 mg, 50 count bottle, OTC. Recall # D-723-2010;

10) Tylenol PM (Acetaminophen/Diphenhydramine HCl) Gelcaps, Extra Strength, Rapid Release, 500 mg/25 mg, 20 count, OTC, NDC 50580-244-20, UPC 3 0045-0244-208. Recall # D-724-2010
CODE
1) Lot Number: AFA060, Exp. Date: 4/30/2012;

2) a) Lot number: ACA003 Exp. Date: 11/30/2011 b) Lot number: ACA002 Exp. Date: 9/30/2011;

3) a) Lot number: ABA567 Exp. Date: 12/31/2010 b) Lot number: ABA574 Exp. Date: 10/31/2010;

4) a) Lot number: ABA005 Exp. Date: 11/30/2010 b) Lot number: ASA206 Exp. Date: 10/31/2011;

5) Lot number: ABA544, Exp. Date: 11/30/2010;

6) a) Lot number: ABA 566, Exp, Date: 11/30/2010, b) Lot number: ACA025, Exp. Date: 12/31/2012, c) Lot number: AFA018, Exp. Date: 4/30/2013, d) Lot number: ABA168, Exp. Date: 11/30/2012;

7) a) Lot number: AJA119, Exp, Date: 6/30/2011 b) Lot number: ACA024, Exp. Date: 12/31/2010;

8) Lot number: ACA005, Exp. Date: 1/31/2011, Lot number: ADA259, Exp. Date: 2/28/2011, Lot number: AEC005, Exp. Date: 1/31/2011, Lot number: AFC005, Exp. Date: 11/30/2010, Lot number: ADC002, Exp. Date: 10/31/2010;

9) Lot number: AFA100, Exp. Date: 4/30/2011;

10) Lot number: ACA004, Exp. Date: 12/31/2010

RECALLING FIRM/MANUFACTURER

Recalling Firm: Mcneil Consumer Healthcare, Div Of Mcneil-ppc, Inc., Fort Washington, PA, by Media, Internet, Fax & Mail beginning July 8, 2010.

Manufacturer: McNeil Healthcare, LLC, Las Piedras, PR. Firm initiated recall is ongoing.

REASON

Chemical Contamination: presence of a chemical called 2,4,6-tribromoanisole (TBA) in products.

VOLUME OF PRODUCT IN COMMERCE

2.468,496 bottles

DISTRIBUTION

Nationwide, Caribbean locations including Trinidad& Tobago, Dominican Republic, Jamaica, Fiji and Guatemal

---

PRODUCT

1) Benadryl (Diphenhydramine HCl) Allergy Ultratabs, 25 mg each, 100 Ultratab bottle, OTC. Recall # D-725-2010;

2) Tylenol Extra Strength Rapid Release Gels (Acetaminophen), 24 and

225 count bottles. Recall # D-726-2010

CODE

1) Lot # AJA008, ABA022, ABA264, ADA194;

2) Lot # ASA202 Expiration date 10/2011

RECALLING FIRM/MANUFACTURER

McNeil Consumer Products Co., Fort Washington, PA, by Media, Internet, Fax & Mail beginning June 8, 2010.

Manufacturer: McNeil Healthcare, LLC, Las Piedras, PR. Firm initiated recall is ongoing.

REASON

Chemical contamination: presence of a chemical called 2,4,6,-tribromoanisole.

VOLUME OF PRODUCT IN COMMERCE

1) 333,288 bottles; 2) 132,120 bottles

DISTRIBUTION

Nationwide, Bermuda, Trinidad and Tobago

The products listed in this recall are household names; drugs that have used by American consumers for years, some of which are manufactured for consumption by children. Any company that suffers from this magnitude of regulatory problems will have a long road back to regaining the trust of consumers, and FDA.

Now before we go any further, so everyone understands what has been presented in terms of recalls, let's clarify some of the not-so-obvious terms used in Table 2 and simplify what triggers a recall.

- Drug application—Many drugs such as new drugs or generics must have FDA approval of their drug application before they can manufacture or distribute that drug for sale. Selling such drugs without an approved drug application is a violation of the law. Many recalls result from this violation.
- cGMP conformance—As mentioned earlier, a drug that is not manufactured under GMPs, even if it meets all of its specifications, may not be released to commerce. Such batches of drugs are subject to recall or seizure.

- Stability failure—drugs are given their shelf lives based upon laboratory experiments known as stability studies. One or more lots of a drug product, in its commercial container (the container that is on the store shelf), are placed into a chamber whose temperature and humidity are carefully controlled within a very narrow range. For a two-year shelf life, the product is tested after 3, 6, 9, 12, 18 and 24 months. If it meets all its specifications at each interval over the 24 month period, it earns a two-year shelf life. Each year one lot of each product in each of its commercial containers is put up on stability. If any of the test intervals (3, 6, 9, 12, 18 or 24 months) produce test results that are out of specification, the lot must be recalled due to a stability failure. **Note:** A failure at 24 months is moot.
- Dissolution—Dissolution is a test that simulates how fast a drug dissolves in one's stomach or intestines. It uses a special piece of equipment that is called, of all things, a dissolution apparatus. Many drug products, particularly tablets and capsules, have a dissolution specification requirement. If a stability sample fails dissolution, the lot gets recalled.
- Sub-potent—Too little active ingredient.
- Super-potent—Too much active ingredient.
- Adverse event—There is a system by which any consumer can report an adverse drug event to a drug manufacturer or to their pharmacist or directly to FDA. After notification of an adverse event, the firm must report it to FDA within three business days. Adverse events, depending upon their seriousness, may result in a recall other action.
- Efficacy—If a drug fails efficacy, it means that it is not effective, that is doesn't work the way it's supposed to.
- Sterility—Products such as injectables or drug preparation for the eyes need to be sterile. Sterility failure equals recall.
- Uniformity—Drug products are expected to be uniform in character. For example, tablets in a batch of drug

product should each be the same weight, thickness and have the same amount of active ingredient and the same dissolution characteristics. Uniformity problems can result in recalls.

- Impurities—All active ingredients have impurities that are supposed to be there, but in limited amounts. If an active ingredient that fails impurity specifications is used in a drug product, that product will be subject to a recall.
- Degradation products—Over time, during a drug's shelf life, breakdown products may form. These must be controlled and must stay within specifications.

It never ceases to amaze me how many regulatory problems exist in the pharmaceutical industry, particularly with generic companies. Despite the process of FDA inspection and despite the consequences of poor regulatory compliance, many company managers, and company executives as well, are still standing around with their heads in the sand hoping that GMP problems will go away by themselves.

Our next chapter, "Drug Approvals and The Generic World", in addition to presenting a detailed look into generic drugs, will further delineate the material presented in this chapter.

CHAPTER THREE

DRUG APPROVALS AND THE GENERIC WORLD

Generics are cheaper than brand name drugs and for that reason are preferred by many consumers and by most health insurance plans. Health plans use what is called a formulary where drugs are divided into five tiers. Tier one, the cheapest, is for preferred generics. Tier two, three and four are for non-preferred generics, preferred brand and non-preferred brand drugs respectively. Tier five is usually reserved for specialty drugs. The higher the tier number, the higher your out of pocket cost. For example, where one might pay eighty or ninety dollars for a 90-day supply of a brand drug (Tier 3), the equivalent generic (Tier 1) might cost less than ten dollars. Are generics really as "good", or do they just plain suck. The answer is "it depends".

Let's start our journey down the generic trail by looking at how prescription drugs are approved by FDA for sale in the United States. We'll discuss OTC drugs later on in the chapter. The drug approval process is long, arduous and very expensive. It's even more expensive when one considers the fact that only a small percentage of new drugs actually make it to market. To bring a new drug to market in the United States is no easy task. Here's how it generally works.

Brand Name (Innovator) Drugs

Suppose we come up with a new molecule that we think might be effective against some serious disease (or any disease for that matter). We first need to do animal studies in order to get some safety data. Then, before starting testing on human subjects or volunteers, we need to file an Investigational New Drug Application (IND) with the FDA. The IND must be approved before any human clinical trials begin. IND applications are defined in federal regulations, which specifies what they must contain. Clinical studies are carried out by a sponsor who can be an individual such as a physician, or a pharmaceutical company.

As stated in the regulations, an IND may be submitted for one or more phases of an investigation. The clinical investigation of a previously untested drug is generally divided into three phases.

Phase 1 includes the initial introduction of an investigational new drug into humans. Phase 1 studies are typically closely monitored and may be conducted in patients or normal volunteer subjects. These studies are designed to determine the metabolism and pharmacologic actions of the drug in humans, the side effects associated with increasing doses, and, if possible, to gain early evidence of effectiveness. During Phase 1, sufficient information about the drug's pharmacokinetics and pharmacological effects, how it acts in the body, should be obtained to permit the design of well-controlled, scientifically valid, Phase 2 studies. The total number of subjects and patients included in Phase 1 studies varies with the drug, but is generally in the range of 20 to 80. Phase 1 also include studies of drug metabolism, structure-activity relationships, and mechanism of action in humans, as well as studies in which investigational drugs are used as research tools to explore biological phenomena or disease processes.

Phase 2 includes the controlled clinical studies conducted to evaluate the effectiveness of the drug for a particular indication or indications in patients with the disease or condition under study and to determine the common short-term side effects and risks associated with the drug. Phase 2 studies are typically well controlled, closely monitored, and conducted in a relatively small number of patients, usually involving no more than several hundred subjects.

Phase 3 studies are expanded controlled and uncontrolled trials. They are performed after preliminary evidence suggesting effectiveness of the drug has been obtained, and are intended to gather the additional information about effectiveness and safety that is needed to evaluate the overall benefit-risk relationship of the drug and to provide an adequate basis for physician labeling. Phase 3 studies usually include from several hundred to several thousand subjects.

The IND application must contain the following general categories of information:

- *Animal Pharmacology and Toxicology*
- *Chemistry and Manufacturing*
- Clinical Protocols *and Investigator Information*

FDA has published guidances for GMP requirements related to INDs for various phases of clinical trials. There is one guidance for INDs for Phase 1 and another that addresses Phase 2 and Phase 3. GMP requirements are less stringent for Phase 1, evolving into full cGMP compliance requirements by time Phase 3 is reached.

The cost of the whole process from drug discovery, preclinical and clinical studies, plus manufacturing and chemistry controls can cost tens of millions to hundreds of millions of dollars or more.

But wait, we're not done yet. Assuming everything goes well, and Phase 3 clinical trials are successful, the next step is to file a New Drug Application (NDA). The NDA is the life story of the drug and must be approved by FDA before the drug can be marketed in the United States.

An NDA contains a number of sections such as chemistry, manufacturing controls (CMC), non-clinical pharmacology and toxicology, human pharmacokinetics and bioavailability, microbiology, clinical data, and statistics. Each of these sections is in itself very detailed. It is not unusual for an NDA to contain half a dozen or more thick volumes of information. Once FDA approves the application, including a preapproval inspection (PAI), the drug can finally be distributed to market.

The bottom line is that the brand name company, more commonly referred to as the innovator, must demonstrate with clinical and toxicological data that a new drug is both safe and effective, and that it is manufactured under full GMP compliance. This includes activities such as setting specifications for ingredients as well as the actual drug product, developing and validating test methods, stability studies, proper packaging and labeling control and appropriate quality oversight. Those six systems we spoke about earlier must all be in full GMP compliance.

OK, can everyone see why innovator (brand name) prescription drugs are so damned expensive? Not only does the innovator spends tens or hundreds of millions of dollars or more to get just one NDA approved, they also have invested in drugs that didn't make it—lots of money down the drain. As an example, not too long ago, a drug for Alzheimer's disease failed Phase 3 clinical trials, resulting in a disastrous loss of an investment rumored to be in the neighborhood of about one billion dollars. The company involved was all geared up to start production and to hire additional people, all for naught.

The innovator, in addition to the financial burden of bringing a new drug to market, has patent protection for only a limited number of years. Generic equivalents cannot be marketed until after the innovator's patent protection expires. So, innovators have only a finite time in which to reap the financial rewards of selling an approved new drug.

Yes, prescription drugs are expensive, some are very expensive, but keep in mind that drug companies are businesses that are expected to be profitable, and like any other business, have to answer to investors and stockholders. If these companies can't make money, they can't continue the research and development needed to come up with new medicines. They can't maintain a pipeline of new drugs.

In addition to the long and expensive drug approval process, once an NDA is approved and the drug goes to market, there are requirements for post-approval surveillance. This includes filing an annual report that includes information on manufacturing (number of lots produced), batch failures, deviations, test data, stability data, complaints, statistical analysis, recalls, adverse events, returns and more.

Hey, but what about us poor patients. We can't always afford some of these drugs, even if we need them, and during the innovator's patent protection period, there are no generic versions legally available, at least here in the United States.

Well, while some think of innovators are "the big bad wolves" whose attitude is "If you can't afford our drugs, tough shit", this is not the case. Prescription drug prices are high for reasons already explained, however, there is no reason anyone should go without needed medications, and you don't have to. For those who have health insurance, no problem. For those who do not, for financial reasons, there are many state programs that provide for prescription drug assistance. As an example, one of my own family members is on total disability due to a serious medical condition. Through state prescription drug assistance, he gets his seven hundred dollar a month medicine for three dollars a month. The programs are out there, just look for them. Don't blame the drug companies, without them, many of us who enjoy active, healthy lives, would be dead and buried. My own father, who died of a heart attack at age 63, would be alive today if he had access to modern medicines. I'm still alive because of today's modern medicines. I always say; "better living through chemistry".

The process of getting a new drug approved in the United States is extremely rigorous and demanding. There is a tremendous burden on drug companies to show that drugs are safe and effective and that the benefits outweigh the risks. Yet, even with the vigorous drug approval process, some medications cause serious health problems after they have been approved, and have to provide additional warnings on the label, a process known as black boxing. In some cases, problems are so severe that the drug is withdrawn from the market. These are the exception rather than the rule. Most drugs approved by FDA safe and effective, within their prescribed limits.

There are a number of prescription drugs that are approved in Europe but not in the United States, and many consumers find ways to get these in lieu of waiting for FDA to approve the drug here at home—not recommended. One example, the diet drug

Acomplia™ (Rimonabant) works great for losing weight. It was approved in Europe, but FDA failed to approve the drug NDA in the United States due to potential serious side effects, even though it passed phase 3 clinical trials. One individual I know bought the drug from England, took it for four months and lost a significant amount of weight. The serious negative neurological side effects suffered by that individual were not worth the weight loss. In general, if FDA rejects a drug, don't look elsewhere for it. This includes on-line and Canadian pharmacy purchases.

GENERICS

OK, now an innovator's patent is about to expire. The generic companies are starting to circle the wagons like a pack of hungry vultures waiting to file a generic drug application.

So, what does a company have to do to market a generic version of a prescription drug? They have to file an Abbreviated New Drug Application, more commonly referred to as an ANDA. Approved ANDAs are generally needed for generic versions of prescription drugs and for OTC drugs that used to be prescription drugs, such as cetirizine, ranitidine, loperamide and 200 mg ibuprofen to name a few. The approval route for an ANDA is much shorter and far less expensive than for an NDA. Why?

While an ANDA does require a fair amount of work to get approved, it is nothing compared to that required for an NDA approval. For one thing, the generic company does not have to demonstrate safety or effectiveness. The innovator has already done that at great expense, and once the patent expires, generic ANDA applicants get the benefit of that work for free. In a nutshell, an NDA applicant pays many millions of dollars to prove safety and effectiveness, while an ANDA applicant, because safety and effectiveness was demonstrated in the NDA, pays nothing. Sounds like a sweet deal for the generic company.

Well then, what does the generic company have to do to get an ANDA approved? For one thing, they have to demonstrate chemistry and manufacturing controls that are as stringent as those for an NDA. GMP compliance requirements are the same for everyone. But then, rather than proving safety and effectiveness, the generic ANDA applicant need only demonstrate bioequivalence. This means that the generic drug applicant has to demonstrate that their drug gets into the blood stream in a time and quantity similar to that of the innovator's drug. This is called a bio-study. Whereas clinical studies for an NDA drug can cost hundreds of millions of dollars, a bio-study can often be purchased for a couple of hundred thousand dollars. For better or worse, probably worse, many companies are outsourcing bio-studies to countries like India where they cost much less. Remember what was said earlier? many generic companies are small firms with limited financial resources that are always bargain-hunting. You get what you pay for. And, bioequivalence is not required for all dosage forms. For example, liquid products like oral solutions do not normally require bio-studies.

Later in this chapter we will explain how bioequivalence studies are conducted and how generic companies cheat the study (load the dice) to enhance their chances of success. Does this mean that a generic drug that's on the market may not be equivalent to its brand name counterpart? You bet!

But first, let's go through the ANDA process of just how a generic drug might get approved, using the tablet dosage form as an example. Let's call our fictitious company SGF (Small Generic Firm). SGF knows a major name brand prescription drug will be coming off patent in six months and decides to develop a generic knockoff (equivalent substitute) and submit an ANDA to FDA for review and approval. They are in race with other generic companies to be first to get their ANDA approved. First one approved gets 180 days exclusivity, where only they can sell the generic drug. After 180 days, anyone with an approved ANDA can jump into the market.

OK, having made the decision to go forward, SGF gets samples of the innovator product, and assigns its formulation scientists the task of coming up with a formula for a generic equivalent that has similar characteristics, mainly, the generic must have the same amount of active ingredient as the innovator's product and it must be bioequivalent. Before proceeding though, SGF must first select a supplier of the active ingredient, and must make sure that the process their prospective supplier uses to manufacture the active ingredient does not infringe upon the patent of another manufacturer of the same active ingredient that is being used in the innovator's product. Let's leave that up to company lawyers. Once the patent search has been conducted and everything looks good, the project can go full-steam ahead.

Once the new generic drug has been formulated a number of things need to be done. SGF must write batch records, step by step instructions for manufacturing the generic drug product. This includes dispensing of ingredients, blending, granulation and compression (making the tablets). Specifications and test need to be developed for each ingredient, both active and non-active, for in-process samples such as blends and for the finished drug product. Here again, the generic firm often gets to use free information that is already available.

There is an official publication called the United States Pharmacopeia (USP). It contains specifications and test methods for hundreds of active and inactive ingredients, and finished drug products. Chances are the specifications and test methods needed by SGF will be found in the USP. If not, SGF will have to develop its own test procedures and specifications.

Test methods must be validated or qualified, depending on whether or not they are USP methods. Validation is simply demonstrating by laboratory studies that a test method is suitable for its intended use. In addition to test methods, manufacturing cleaning procedures and manufacturing process themselves must be validated. It must be demonstrated through validation studies that cleaning procedures are effective in removing residual drugs and residual detergents from manufacturing equipment. In addition, manufacturing process validation provides a high degree of assurance that the manufacturing process can consistently produce product that meets its predetermined quality attributes (specifications).

Now that we have the chemistry and manufacturing sections which include raw material, in-process and finished product specifications and validated test methods, plus cleaning and process validation, let's move onto drug stability.

All ANDAs, like NDAs, must include stability data. What's that? Have you ever wondered how shelf life of a drug product is determined? Is shelf life plucked out of the air or is it based upon sound scientific studies? The answer is drug stability studies. A drug product in its actual commercial package (the package that you see on the store shelf) is placed into a chamber that is controlled at 40 degrees Celsius and 75 percent relative humidity (accelerated stability) for a period of three months. Samples are removed and tested at one, two and three months. If after three months, the drug product continues to meet its specifications, the drug can be given a <u>predicted</u> two-year shelf life. This must be verified by conducting a real time stability study; placing samples of drug product in a chamber controlled at 25 degrees Celsius and 60 percent relative humidity for two years. Samples are withdrawn and tested at three, six, nine, twelve, eighteen and twenty four months. If each interval meets specifications, then the two year shelf life is confirmed. Stability testing is done using test methods that have been specially validated for use with these samples. These methods can tell if the active ingredient still meets specifications at each test interval and how much it has degraded. Some drug products don't degrade at all, while others do, sometimes significantly. Only the accelerated three-month data is needed for submitting an ANDA for approval. Once approved, the drug can marketed with only the accelerated stability information available at the time of approval. *Stability studies for different types of products can vary, but this is fundamentally how it's normally done.*

So now SGF has demonstrated that they make the product under cGMP conditions, and that drug stability is good. Now it's time for bioequivalence, an area that is wide open to cheating and fudging. Oh boy!

In order for a generic drug to be approved, the generic drug company, in this case our friend SGF, must show that the generic drug is bioequivalent to the innovator's drug. The first step is to run what is known as dissolution profiles. This is a test that simulates how a drug dissolves in the stomach over time. It is done using a piece of equipment called a dissolution apparatus. A typical dissolution unit is shown below.

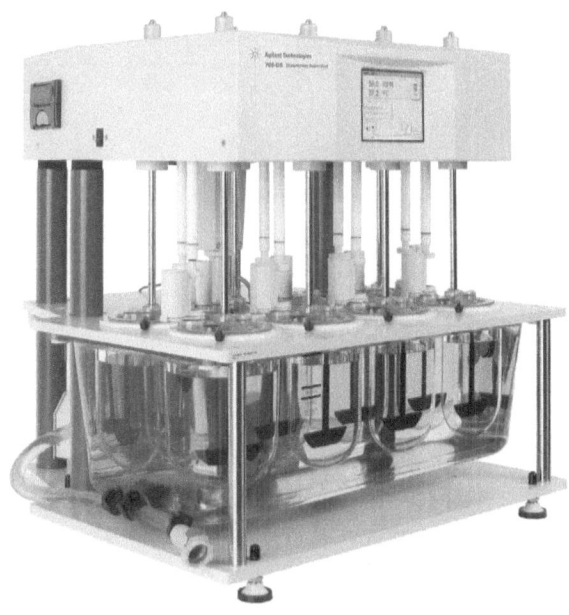

Figure 1
Courtesy of Agilent Technologies

Each glass vessel holds a solution such as simulated gastric fluid or a buffer of some kind. The volume of fluid is just under one liter which is the approximate volume of a person's stomach. To run the test, a single tablet is dropped into each vessel and the paddles are turned on to rotate at a certain speed. The temperature is 37 degrees Celsius which is human body temperature. A small but exact amount of liquid is withdrawn at different time intervals and measured for the amount of active drug that has dissolved. A typical profile might be 5, 10, 20 and 30 minutes. There are other possible combinations such as 15, 30, 45 and 60 minutes. It is beyond the scope of this book to go into how those intervals are picked. The important thing is to match the generic profile as closely as possible to the innovator's profile. Then we plot time versus percent drug dissolved and we get what is called a dissolution profile. The profile is usually done using twelve tablets, so we need two dissolution machines. A typical profile is shown below.

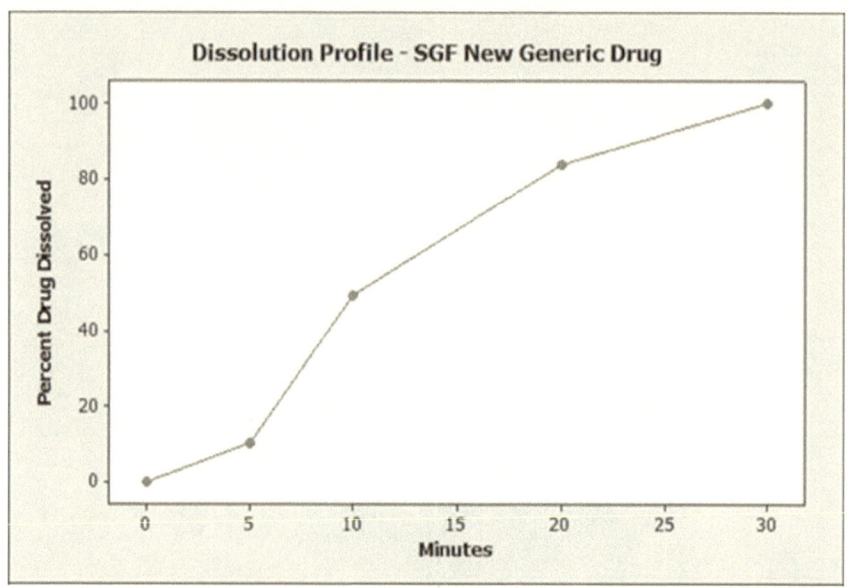

Figure 2

This one shows us that all 12 tablets behave about the same and that at 5 minutes around ten percent of the drug has dissolved, at 10 minutes about 50 percent, at 20 minutes about 85 percent and at 30 minutes close to100 percent.

So now, in order to load the gun for success, SGF runs dissolution profiles on their product along with different lots of the innovators' product, and picks the innovator's lot that most closely matches their generic version. When the ANDA is submitted, a bottle of innovator drug and the generic drug must each be submitted to FDA. Holy, cow, SGF picks what lot of innovator drug they get to compare themselves to. How about that? The generic company can hand pick which lot of innovator's drug they want to use for their bio-study as a comparison to theirs. Talk about stacking the deck?

Now SGF will fiddle around until they can find a lot of the innovator's drug whose dissolution profile closely matches that of its own generic version.

OK, now we have a close match. These are the two lots (one innovator and one generic) that will be submitted for the bio-study. Remember, these studies can run a couple of hundred thousand dollars or more, so SGF must try to load the dice in order to increase the odds that their drug will pass the first time around. They did this by hand-picking a lot of innovator's drug whose dissolution profile closely matched that of its own generic drug.

The way a bio-study generally works, is that the drug is first tried on a small group of patients as a fasting study (no eating for 12 hours before the study). The fasting study is a trial balloon that isn't prohibitively expensive. If the fasting study passes, then it's full steam ahead with the full study which involves many more patients and includes food challenge experiments where patients eat a fatty meal for example before the study. If the drug passes the complete bio-study, we are almost home free. Bio-studies are generally conducted by contract research organization (CROs) that have the appropriate clinical settings to dose and monitor patients, and who have the laboratory facilities and special test methods needed to run accurate analyses on blood samples. Development and validation of these bioanalytical test methods, if not available, are paid for by the generic drug company, in this case our friends at SGF.

So what does passing a bio-study actually entail? Well, the way it works is that patients are given the drug, then blood samples are taken every so often to see how much drug is in the blood stream at that point in time. Samples are taken until the drug concentration peaks in the blood and then until the drug levels in the blood have returned to nominally zero. A curve is plotted of time versus drug concentration in the blood. It might look like the graph shown in Figure 3.

Patients are dosed with the generic drug and with the innovator drug that SGF submitted for the study. If the maximum concentration of drug in the blood and the area under the curve of the generic is within 20 percent of the values for the innovator, the generic passes the bioequivalence portion of the generic approval process. If the generic doesn't pass, SGF will have to reformulate to come with a version of their drug that does pass. Failing and retrying is quite expensive and is therefore avoided if possible. That's why they cheat (sort of).

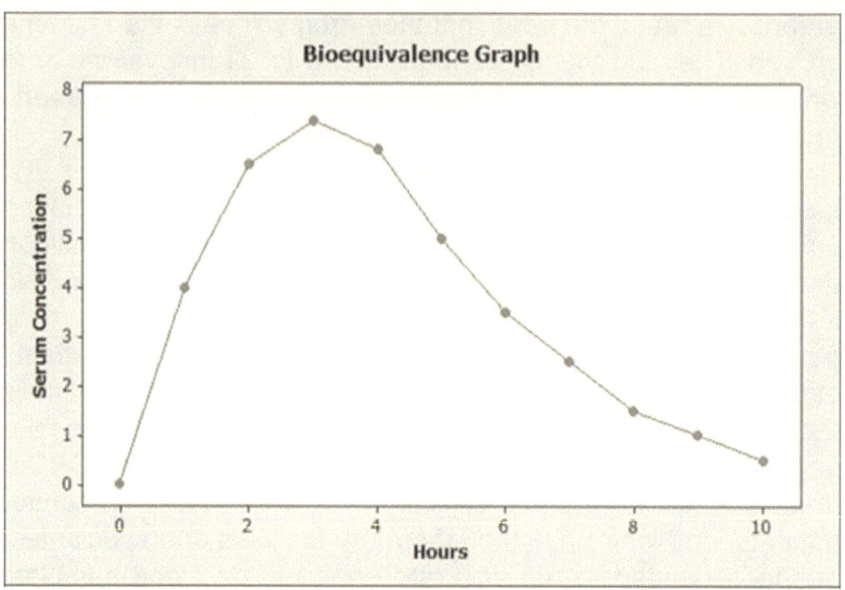

Figure 3

If the bioequivalence passes, does that mean the generic releases active ingredient into your bloodstream the same way as the brand drug?—maybe not. The only thing for sure is that the lot of brand drug that was hand-picked by SGF, behaves the same as the lot of generic drug that was hand-picked by SGF. It doesn't mean that a typical lot of SGF's generic will behave in the body that same way as a typical lot of the innovators' drug. An example is the blood thinner Coumadin (warfarin). The brand and generic, allegedly the same, behave differently in the body. By the way, warfarin is also used as rat poison. Anybody want a piece of cheese?

Now that everything seems to be in order, it's time for SGF to file the ANDA with FDA. Once it is approved, and the innovator's patent protection has expired, SGF can start selling the new generic drug right away. What a break for consumers, right?—maybe. Generic companies are often far from being saints when it comes to helping consumers save money. One example is a generic cancer drug that was approved in the early 1990s. The innovator (brand) sold for $4.00 per tablet. The new generic version sold for $2.70 per tablet.....My hero? Bullshit— the drug cost only eleven cents per tablet to manufacture. So while some generics are actually much cheaper than the innovator's drug, some are not. One up side of generic approvals is that competition is increased, so everyone, including the innovator, tends to start lowering prices.

GENERIC Rx vs.OTCs

There are many good reputable generic manufacturers out there, but with that being said, why do I, this author, in most instances still prefer the brand name drugs over generics?, particularly with over the counter (OTC) drugs. There are a number of reasons.

I worry less about prescription generics because these drug need to have an approved abbreviated new drug application (ANDA) before they can be distributed for sale in the United States. Also, there are some built-in safeguards. As already mentioned, ANDA requirements from the standpoint of manufacturing, testing, drug stability, and quality oversight are subject to the same rigid standards as those required for innovator (brand name) drugs. In addition, generic drugs that have an approved ANDA, are subject to the same post-market surveillance requirements as their brand name counterparts.

So, our company SGF, like every other generic firm with an approved ANDA, must file an annual report, usually on the anniversary of their ANDA approval. An annual report must be filed for each and every approved ANDA generic drug. As with NDA (brand name) drugs, the annual report must contain certain information such as a review of all batches made, manufacturing, packaging and labeling performance, complaints, returns, material destroyed, yield, adverse events, stability and test data for both finished product and active ingredients, and, a statistical analysis of process performance that demonstrates whether or not the manufacturing process for the drug is under control, more specifically, that the manufacturing process will produce product that consistently, lot by lot, meets all its predetermined quality attributes. In laymen's terms, is every lot of generic drug the same quality?

Another safeguard is the choice of active ingredient supplier. The suppliers of all raw materials used for an ANDA-approved generic drugs must actually be listed in the ANDA itself. This means that all the manufacturing, testing, stability and bioequivalence work is conducted using the listed active ingredients. Any post-approval modifications to the ANDA such as manufacturing process changes, specification changes, test method changes, shelf-life extensions, scale up in batch size or change in a raw material supplier must be pre-approved by FDA. For changing or adding an active ingredient supplier, much of the work done for the original ANDA submission and approval must be repeated, using generic drug made with the new supplier's active ingredient. This work may include new process and test method validation studies and stability studies, plus an evaluation of impurities associated with the new active ingredient, and perhaps even bioequivalence.

Going forward we will refer to active ingredients as APIs (active pharmaceutical ingredient). Different manufacturers use different chemical processes to make their APIs, thus each API will have an impurity profile associated with its particular chemical process. Remember, drug products are made by mixing things together while APIs are made using chemical reactions. Even if the API supplier listed in the ANDA changes their process, additional work on the ANDA generic drug may be required.

In order for SGF to sell product made with a different API, they must file what is called a PAS (preapproval supplement). FDA will review the data and then decide whether to approve or not approve the PAS. SGF cannot sell drug product made with the new API without a PAS approval.

Let's assume that the PAS gets approved. Now we have a generic drug that is made under GMPs, has good stability, whose test methods work and whose manufacturing process is validated. And, SGF can use any one of two approved API suppliers. Sounds good, right?

Stop the presses, what about bioequivalence? Remember we suggested that a typical lot of generic drug may or may not release API into your body the same way as a typical lot of the brand name drug? What about a generic drug that uses more than one API supplier. Wow, not only do we have to worry about comparison to the brand name drug, but whether or not the generic drug made with the original API behaves the same as generic drug made with the new API.

Once again, citing the example of warfarin, only you and your doctor can make an informed decision about the benefits of generics versus brand name drugs. For me personally, the only advantage of generic prescription drugs is price, although as previously mentioned, there are a number of reputable generic drug companies. I plead guilty, from time to time, of having used prescription generics manufactured by some of those reputable companies such as Mylan and Teva. Finally, in fairness to manufacturers of prescription generic drugs, many are fine in both quality and performance. My main concern is with lot-to-lot bioequivalence versus innovator product, especially when it comes to extended-release products.

GENERIC OTCs

Now the real fun begins. While generic prescription drugs tend to be generally safe and effective , although I do have concerns about bioequivalence, and are manufactured and monitored with the same scrutiny as NDA (brand name) drugs, the OTC world is totally, totally, totally different. Buyer beware!

Over the counter (OTC) drugs, with the exception of those that used to be prescription drugs, do not need an approved drug application (ANDA) in order to be put on the market. The only basic requirement for OTCs is that they are manufactured under GMP conditions, and that their ingredients are generally recognized as safe and effective. Remember the example in Chapter One of our fictitious company called "Garage Pharmaceuticals"? Keep that in mind as you read on. The OTC manufacturer can use any API and inactive ingredient suppliers they want and can change suppliers at will to accommodate supply chain and price requirements.

What about those suppliers? Remember, as mentioned earlier, that many generic OTC companies are small ,"mom and pop" type, privately-owned operations where everything is driven by price. So, they often buy the cheapest raw materials, hire the lowest-paid workers, including manufacturing personnel and laboratory chemists, and take every shortcut possible to save a buck or two. Once again what about those suppliers?

The API (active ingredient) that is in the drug product you buy, whether it's a pain-relief tablet or capsule, or a cough syrup for example, should be pure and not adulterated (contaminated) with harmful impurities. When buying an OTC at your local drugstore or supermarket, you shouldn't have to worry about whether or not the product is safe to use. Is it going to help me or hurt me? That's not the question you want to be asking yourself. Well, unfortunately, from time to time, that's exactly the question you might have to ask.

APIs and inactives are manufactured by countries all over the world. There are many foreign countries, from my personal experience, that make high quality chemicals such as Japan, UK, France, Germany, Spain and Italy. Then there is China and India. Materials from these countries are cheap and for my money of relatively poor quality. Guess who the small generic OTC manufacturer, with limited financial resources, is going to go to buy their APIs? That's right, China and India. These APIs are cheap and in my opinion, generally suck. There is a very good chance that store-brand or discount OTC drugs are made using Chinese or Indian raw materials. We'll touch on this again later.

The OTC manufacturer can use any lot of API from any supplier they want, so long as that API meets some minimum uniform standard. Recall earlier we mentioned an official book called the USP that contains specifications and test methods for many active ingredients, inactive ingredients (known as excipients) and finished drug products. Just about every imaginable OTC drug and its ingredients can be found in the USP. Now USP specifications for APIs usually involve requirements for percent purity, identification and other tests such as water content, and some limit test such as heavy metals, or some specific impurity or impurities. If an API is tested using USP test methods and meets all the listed USP specifications, then the API can be released for use in a drug product. But wait, the OTC manufacturer doesn't have to run all the tests every time it receives a lot of that API. The only requirement under GMPS is that the company performs at least one specific identity test in conjunction with receipt of a certificate of analysis. The only additional requirement is that the OTC manufacturer periodically conduct all the tests to verify the certificate of analysis. This is usually done on one to three lots per year. Bottom line; a whole lot of testing doesn't get done—we trust the API supplier's test results. But how reliable are those test results? Can we really trust the API manufacturer? Well, that depends.

Ok, we have tested the API according to USP test methods and all USP specifications have been met. This should give us a high degree of confidence that that API is suitable for use in an OTC drug product. But wait; what if the API is contaminated with something that we are not testing for? Do we take the position that if an API has no USP specification for cyanide content for example, that it's alright for that API to contain cyanide? It is expected that an API manufacturer will supply material that is chemically pure, meets all it specifications is not contaminated with any foreign substance or additive. One cannot always make that assumption.

Ready for this?—Many chemical tests for purity of an API or other chemical used in drug products, or food products for that matter, can be fooled by adding something that makes the purity of the API or other chemical seem higher than it actually is. This can be done because some test methods are not specific enough to detect the difference between contaminated and uncontaminated material. Sometimes a drug or chemical is just plain contaminated. Two glaring example come to mind, both involving material from China.

The first situation involves contaminated glycerin from China. Glycerin is commonly used in pharmaceutical preparations as a sweetener in oral products or as a base in products such as ear drops. FDAs guidance entitled "Testing of Glycerin for Diethylene Glycol" resulted from this problem. Quoting from the Introduction and Background in this guidance:

"This guidance is intended to alert pharmaceutical manufacturers, pharmacy compounders,

repackers, and suppliers to the potential public health hazard of glycerin contaminated with

diethylene glycol (DEG), a poison. FDA has received and continues to receive (most recently in

October 2006) reports about fatal DEG poisoning of consumers who ingested medicinal syrups,

such as cough syrup or acetaminophen syrup, that were manufactured with DEG-contaminated

glycerin. This guidance provides recommendations that will help pharmaceutical manufacturers,

repackers, and other suppliers of glycerin, and pharmacists who engage in drug compounding,

avoid the use of glycerin that is contaminated with DEG and prevent incidents of DEG

poisoning.

"In late 1995 and early 1996, many children were admitted to hospitals in Port-au-Prince, Haiti, with sudden kidney failure, resulting in at least 80 fatalities. An

investigation by Haitian health officials, the Centers for Disease Control (CDC), and FDA

discovered that the cause was DEG-contaminated glycerin in acetaminophen syrup manufactured

in Haiti. Between 1990 and 1998, similar incidents of DEG poisoning occurred in Argentina,

Bangladesh, India, and Nigeria and resulted in the deaths of hundreds of children. In October

2006, an outbreak of DEG poisoning occurred in Panama, resulting in multiple cases of illness

and death".

Now, pharmaceutical companies who use glycerin, before releasing a lot for use in their drug products, must test each individual drum or container for diethylene glycol and for ethylene glycol (a related compound) content. The allowable safe limit is 0.10% maximum of each.

Holy cow! Sure, now we test every container of glycerin. But suppose someone screwed up the test and glycerin with a high diethylene glycol (DEG) or ethylene glycol (EG) content slipped by and was used in a drug product. Just for everyone's information, DEG and EG are main components of automobile antifreeze. Would you want to give your child a cough medicine, or your young infant, eardrops that contain antifreeze. Kind of makes your blood run cold doesn't it? Propylene glycol, a material similar to glycerin used in pharmaceuticals, cosmetics and personal care products is now also required to be tested for DEG and EG content. Getting back to the main point, generic OTCs are often made from cheap ingredients from countries whose regulatory, safety standards and manufacturing controls are not quite up to snuff.

The second example involves a food problem included here to make a further point about the risks of using ingredients from countries like China. Back in 2007, it was found that wheat gluten used in pet food, imported from China, contained melamine, an industrial chemical with a multitude of uses. On March 15, 2007, FDA learned that certain pet foods were sickening and killing cats and dogs. FDA found contaminants in vegetable proteins imported into the United States from China and used as ingredients in pet food. As a result of FDA and USDA's comprehensive investigation, on February 6, 2008, FDA announced that two Chinese nationals and the businesses they operate, along with a U.S. company and its president and chief executive officer, were indicted by a federal grand jury for their roles in a scheme to import products purported to be wheat gluten into the United States that were contaminated with melamine.

Now why would anyone want to add a substance like melamine to a product like wheat gluten? The answer is that the quality of substances like wheat gluten is measured by its protein content, which is in turn determined by testing for percent nitrogen. Chemicals like melamine have a very high nitrogen content, therefore, adding some melamine to the wheat gluten will make it appear much purer than it actually is. Since there is no way to know from a simple nitrogen content test that there is anything wrong, spiking the product with melamine was a neat way to cheat and commit fraud. Too bad lots of pets had to die to find out which bottom-feeding low-lives were responsible. Since then, a number of pharmaceutical ingredients including common additives like lactose and gelatin have been identified as being at risk for melamine contamination. Now, as a result, drug companies need to comply with FDA Guidance for Industry, "Pharmaceutical Components at Risk for Melamine Contamination"

So, let's buy American. Take acetaminophen for example, the active ingredient in Tylenol®. Almost every OTC manufacturer and their mother makes acetaminophen-containing products ranging from tablets, capsules and oral solutions and suspensions containing acetaminophen alone or in combination with other drugs. Acetaminophen concentrations in drug products are quite high, usually 325 milligrams or 500 milligrams per unit dose. There are two impurities in acetaminophen that must be tested for, to make sure that they are each below a certain limit. If one purchases acetaminophen from a major American manufacturer, the material will usually be snow-white in appearance and contain little or no measurable impurities. On the other hand, material from places like China and India will have an off-white or yellowish appearance and contain measurable amounts of its two major impurities, often at levels that are close to the allowable upper limit. Both materials meet USP specifications and can therefore be used in a drug product. Are both materials of equal quality? If one defines quality as conformance to specifications, then the answer is yes, but the grade is certainly not the same. Why buy the material that looks yellowish and barely meets specifications for impurity limits? The answer with generic OTC manufacturers as always is price.

Now let's get back on track. As we started to say, generic OTC manufacturers can use whatever sources of ingredients they want so long as these materials meet certain minimum uniform standards such as USP specifications. Not to beat a dead horse, but the decision on what to buy is usually price-driven. OK, so generic OTCs are often made with the cheapest ingredients that are barely acceptable from a quality standpoint.

The generic OTC market is brutally competitive. For a generic OTC manufacturer to make money, they have to sell their products in volume, usually at relatively low prices. Typical outlets are discount chains such as Dollar Tree. Even when the generic OTC company gets into bigger chains such as Wal-Mart or Target, price pressure continues to persist. Many generic OTC companies are small with less than 10 million dollars a year in sales. The best they can hope for is to get into a major drug chain like CVS or Walgreens, and ultimately, get their own ANDA approved and have a branded product under their own name. Generally though, these small companies just muddle through with minimal sales to discount-type customers, using marginally acceptable ingredients and cutting corners wherever possible to make a buck.

When you as a consumer go into a drug store, discount store or supermarket and decide to buy the store brand of a drug, you can't be sure where the ingredients came from, whether or not the product was properly manufactured or tested for quality, or whether or not it will remain good over time (drug stability).

Now don't get me wrong. Major drug chains like CVS and Walgreens have very high quality standards and do check out their suppliers or prospective suppliers by sending in their own auditors and by using consumer panels to evaluate things such as taste, odor and appearance. However, you can't watch everything all the time, plus the generic OTC manufacturer still picks their own suppliers and may well continue to cut corners as needed to make money.

Store brand and private label OTC products are almost always made by generic OTC contract manufacturers. What's that? Contract manufacturers are companies that make other company's drugs. Why would a company hire another company to make its product? There are several possibilities. First, the contracting company may not have the capacity and therefore farms out some of the work. Another scenario that is becoming more prevalent is the virtual company. There are a number of virtual companies that don't make anything themselves. They own ANDAs, and even have their own brands, but make nothing themselves. Everything is farmed out from manufacturing, packaging, labeling and distribution. The only thing the virtual company might have is sales, marketing, administration, legal, finance, regulatory and quality. Some of these companies are very successful, running 100 or 200 million dollar a year operations out of an office building with a small staff. The virtual company has the responsibility of monitoring and auditing all of their contact organizations to assure proper GMP compliance and suitable quality standards.

Even some large brand-name companies farm out manufacturing, however, these larger companies from my experience, tend to be more vigilant in their oversight of contract organizations.

Contract work is hard to manage. There is contract manufacturing, contract packaging and labeling, plus contract chemical and microbiological testing. Just about every aspect of pharmaceutical manufacturing and quality control can be farmed out. Manufacturing can be subdivided where one contactor makes a blend (drug intermediate) and a different contractor compresses the tablets. It's a lot to handle and things can go wrong.

For me, in most cases, more expensive or not, it's buy the brand name OTC drug. If I have a headache, it's Bayer® aspirin, not the store brand. If I have an allergy, it's Benadryl®, not the store brand and so on. But that's just me. The choice is yours.

Generic OTCs are supposed to be equivalent to the brand just as generic prescription products are supposed to be equivalent to the brand. So let's see; are generic OTC products and brand name OTCs bioequivalent? Who knows, since no bioequivalence studies were ever conducted. For solid dosages such as tablets and capsules, is generic OTC tablet to tablet or capsule to capsule uniformity as good as that for the brand OTC? Is the generic OTC formulated to assure that the active ingredient is always at 100 percent of stated label claim? Active ingredient specifications for drug products is generally 90 to 110 percent of label claim. For example, for a 500 milligram aspirin tablets, any aspirin levels between 450 and 550 milligrams per tablet would meet specifications. The regulations state that a drug manufacturer's process must target 100 percent of label claim. But what if the generic company, for money reasons or just to screw the consumer, decided to produce tablets or capsules that routinely assayed at about 97 percent of label claim—in the case of our aspirin tablet, you as the consumer would be paying for 500 milligram of aspirin per tablet but would be getting on average only 485 milligrams of aspirin per tablet. No big deal, or is it. Aspirin is cheap and the therapeutic difference between 485 milligrams and 500 milligrams is insignificant. But what if an expensive active ingredient was involved whose dosing level was important? Once again, brand OTC or generic OTC? The choice is yours.

One final piece of information on non-prescription drugs; there used to be just prescription drugs and over the counter drugs, Rx or OTC. Now there is another category called BTC, behind the counter drugs. These are non-prescription drugs that are kept behind the counter and issued by a pharmacist in limited quantities only. Certain active ingredients such as pseudoephedrine, a common decongestant, can be easily converted to an illegal controlled substance methamphetamine. Products containing actives such as pseudoephedrine are dispensed without a prescription, but by a pharmacist in order to control the maximum amount that can be purchased at one time. As with other categories, BTC drugs have brand name and generic versions. The issues discussed for generic OTC drugs apply to generic BTC drugs as well.

Dietary Supplements (Nutraceuticals)

Nutritional supplements, also known as nutraceuticals, have recently come under strict regulation in a manner analogous to that used for drug products. Drug GMPs are defined in the Code of Federal Regulations, Title 21, Part 211 (21 CFR 211). The new nutritional supplement GMPS are cited in the Code of Federal Regulations, Title 21, Part 111 (21 CFR 111), entitled "CURRENT GOOD MANUFACTURING PRACTICE IN MANUFACTURING, PACKAGING, LABELING, OR HOLDING OPERATIONS FOR DIETARY SUPPLEMENTS". Since nutraceutical products are over the counter (OTC) items, and mostly generic, they are included in this chapter and are considered generic drugs.

Prior to being regulated, nutritional supplements were generally classified as foods instead of drugs. When FDA inspected a company that manufactured both drugs and nutritional supplements, they would do a thorough inspection of the drug manufacturing operations for GMP compliance, but would pretty much ignore nutritional supplements because they were thought of as a food product. Even vitamins were classified as foods. Not only that, no regulations existed for nutritional supplements against which to audit or inspect. Now, we not only have GMPs for nutraceuticals, we have official test methods and specifications listed in the USP. Yes, now the USP contains specifications and test methods for active drug ingredients, inactive drug ingredients, drug products and nutraceuticals. Actually, the USP has always had test methods and specifications for vitamins, even though vitamins in themselves were considered foods.

Nutraceuticals now listed in the USP, for which test methods and specifications are given, include things such as vitamins, amino acids, saw palmetto, ginseng, minerals such as chromium and many, many more. The USP currently lists dozens of dietary supplements along with specifications and test methods. Just about anything that can be purchased in a health food store or a supermarket or drug store's vitamin and dietary supplement section is now included in the USP. An updated, new USP is published yearly, with supplements every four months. Thus information on dietary supplements and drugs are always being added or modified.

So what's the big deal with dietary supplements (nutraceuticals)? How come products that were considered foods, are now regulated in a manner similar to the way drugs are regulated. Dietary supplements aren't drugs are they? Well, in the sense that the dietary supplement manufacturing does not involve taking a pure active drug and formulating it into a tablet, capsule, solution, suspension, cream, ointment, suppository or other dosage form, the answer is no. However, in some cases, dietary supplements are drugs. Many dietary supplements are plant-derived, such as saw palmetto for example. Saw palmetto contains fatty acids plus drugs known as phytosterols. Phyto means from plants, so phytosterols are steroids that are plant-derived.

Some plants do actually contain drugs, yes, drugs do occur in nature in plants. And, there are dietary supplements that contain naturally occurring drugs in the plants from which they are derived. Some can even dangerous if misused. One glaring example that comes to mind is ephedra, also known as ma huang. This dietary supplement which is no longer on the market contained about ten percent ephedrine, which is a very powerful decongestant capable of dangerously raising ones blood pressure. To put things into perspective, a drug product containing ephedrine, or more likely its chemically equivalent first cousin pseudoephedrine, would have a dose of about 30 mg. A 600 milligram tablet for example would contain about five percent drug. But with the ephdra-containing dietary supplement, at ten percent ephedrine and no dosing guidelines, ingestion of ephedrine would typically be much higher. For someone with a heart condition or high blood pressure, ingestion of too much ephedrine could be disastrous. Due to serious side effects and a number of deaths, FDA on April 12, 2004, banned the sale of ephedrine-containing dietary supplements. Because this product was a huge money-maker, manufacturers of ephedra dietary supplements challenged the ban, which was upheld by the U.S. Court of Appeals for the Tenth Circuit in 2006. It is now illegal in the United States to sell ephedra-containing dietary supplements.

As a consultant and contract laboratory owner who has done extensive work with dietary supplements, I can really sympathize with dietary supplement manufactures who have to change their mindsets and way of doing business in order to comply with the new regulations. It used to be that one could order raw materials, whip up a batch, ship it out and count the money. Now, they must operate under dietary supplement GMPs.

These GMPs were published at least two years before becoming official, plenty of time to get ready. The problem is, dietary supplement manufacturers, having had no experience with a GMP operations, were at somewhat of a loss as to how to get ready. We all had to learn together. These new regulations are tough. It's as if FDA took the drug regulations and the food regulations and shuffled them together. Requirements that are routine for drug manufacturing such as validation, testing and quality control responsibilities were suddenly thrust upon the dietary supplement industry.

A copy of the new regulations (21 CFR 111) table of contents is presented below to illustrate just how extensive the new regulations are.

PART 111   CURRENT GOOD MANUFACTURING PRACTICE
IN MANUFACTURING, PACKAGING, LABELING,
OR HOLDING OPERATIONS FOR DIETARY
SUPPLEMENTS

Subpart A--General Provisions

§ 111.1 - *Who is subject to this part?*

§ 111.3 - *What definitions apply to this part?*

§ 111.5 - *Do other statutory provisions and regulations apply?*

Subpart B--Personnel

§ 111.8 - *What are the requirements under this subpart B for written procedures?*

§ 111.10 - *What requirements apply for preventing microbial contamination from sick or infected personnel and for hygienic practices?*

§ 111.12 - *What personnel qualification requirements apply?*

§ 111.13 - *What supervisor requirements apply?*

§ 111.14 - *Under this subpart B, what records must you make and keep?*

Subpart C--Physical Plant and Grounds

§ 111.15 - *What sanitation requirements apply to your physical plant and grounds?*

§ 111.16 - *What are the requirements under this subpart C for written procedures?*

§ 111.20 - *What design and construction requirements apply to your physical plant?*

§ 111.23 - *Under this subpart C, what records must you make and keep?*

Subpart D--Equipment and Utensils

§ 111.25 - *What are the requirements under this subpart D for written procedures?*

§ 111.27 - *What requirements apply to the equipment and utensils that you use?*

§ 111.30 - *What requirements apply to automated, mechanical, or electronic equipment?*

§ 111.35 - *Under this subpart D, what records must you make and keep?*

Subpart E--Requirement to Establish a Production and Process Control System

§ 111.55 - *What are the requirements to implement a production and process control system?*

§ 111.60 - *What are the design requirements for the production and process control system?*

§ 111.65 - *What are the requirements for quality control operations?*

§ 111.70 - *What specifications must you establish?*

§ 111.73 - *What is your responsibility for determining whether established specifications are met?*

§ 111.75 - *What must you do to determine whether specifications are met?*

§ 111.77 - *What must you do if established specifications are not met?*

§ 111.80 - *What representative samples must you collect?*

§ 111.83 - *What are the requirements for reserve samples?*

§ 111.87 - *Who conducts a material review and makes a disposition decision?*

§ 111.90 - *What requirements apply to treatments, in-process adjustments, and reprocessing when there is a deviation or unanticipated occurrence or when a specification established in accordance with 111.70 is not met?*

§ 111.95 - *Under this subpart E, what records must you make and keep?*

Subpart F--Production and Process Control System: Requirements for Quality Control

§ 111.103 - *What are the requirements under this subpart F for written procedures?*

§ 111.105 - *What must quality control personnel do?*

§ 111.110 - *What quality control operations are required for laboratory operations associated with the production and process control system?*

§ 111.113 - *What quality control operations are required for a material review and disposition decision?*

§ 111.117 - *What quality control operations are required for equipment, instruments, and controls?*

§ 111.120 - *What quality control operations are required for components, packaging, and labels before use in the manufacture of a dietary supplement?*

§ 111.123 - *What quality control operations are required for the master manufacturing record, the batch production record, and manufacturing operations?*

§ 111.127 - *What quality control operations are required for packaging and labeling operations?*

§ 111.130 - *What quality control operations are required for returned dietary supplements?*

§ 111.135 - *What quality control operations are required for product complaints?*

§ 111.140 - *Under this subpart F, what records must you make and keep?*

Subpart G--Production and Process Control System: Requirements for Components, Packaging, and Labels and for Product That You Receive for Packaging or Labeling as a Dietary Supplement

§ 111.153 - *What are the requirements under this subpart G for written procedures?*

§ 111.155 - *What requirements apply to components of dietary supplements?*

§ 111.160 - *What requirements apply to packaging and labels received?*

§ 111.165 - *What requirements apply to a product received for packaging or labeling as a dietary supplement (and for distribution rather than for return to the supplier)?*

§ 111.170 - *What requirements apply to rejected components, packaging, and labels, and to rejected products that are received for packaging or labeling as a dietary supplement?*

§ 111.180 - *Under this subpart G, what records must you make and keep?*

Subpart H--Production and Process Control System: Requirements for the Master Manufacturing Record

§ 111.205 - *What is the requirement to establish a master manufacturing record?*

§ 111.210 - *What must the master manufacturing record include?*

Subpart I--Production and Process Control System: Requirements for the Batch Production Record

§ 111.255 - *What is the requirement to establish a batch production record?*

§ 111.260 - *What must the batch record include?*

Subpart J--Production and Process Control System: Requirements for Laboratory Operations

§ 111.303 - *What are the requirements under this subpart J for written procedures?*

§ 111.310 - *What are the requirements for the laboratory facilities that you use?*

§ 111.315 - *What are the requirements for laboratory control processes?*

§ 111.320 - *What requirements apply to laboratory methods for testing and examination?*

§ 111.325 - *Under this subpart J, what records must you make and keep?*

Subpart K--Production and Process Control System: Requirements for Manufacturing Operations

§ 111.353 - *What are the requirements under this subpart K for written procedures?*

§ 111.355 - *What are the design requirements for manufacturing operations?*

§ 111.360 - *What are the requirements for sanitation?*

§ 111.365 - *What precautions must you take to prevent contamination?*

§ 111.370 - *What requirements apply to rejected dietary supplements?*

§ 111.375 - *Under this subpart K, what records must you make and keep?*

Subpart L--Production and Process Control System: Requirements for Packaging and Labeling Operations

§ 111.403 - *What are the requirements under this subpart L for written procedures?*

§ 111.410 - *What requirements apply to packaging and labels?*

§ 111.415 - *What requirements apply to filling, assembling, packaging, labeling, and related operations?*

§ 111.420 - *What requirements apply to repackaging and relabeling?*

§ 111.425 - *What requirements apply to a packaged and labeled dietary supplement that is rejected for distribution?*

§ 111.430 - *Under this subpart L, what records must you make and keep?*

Subpart M--Holding and Distributing

§ 111.453 - *What are the requirements under this subpart for M written procedures?*

§ 111.455 - *What requirements apply to holding components, dietary supplements, packaging, and labels?*

§ 111.460 - *What requirements apply to holding in-process material?*

§ 111.465 - *What requirements apply to holding reserve samples of dietary supplements?*

§ 111.470 - *What requirements apply to distributing dietary supplements?*

§ 111.475 - *Under this subpart M, what records must you make and keep?*

Subpart N--Returned Dietary Supplements

§ 111.503 - *What are the requirements under this subpart N for written procedures?*

§ 111.510 - *What requirements apply when a returned dietary supplement is received?*

§ 111.515 - *When must a returned dietary supplement be destroyed, or otherwise suitably disposed of?*

§ 111.520 - *When may a returned dietary supplement be salvaged?*

§ 111.525 - *What requirements apply to a returned dietary supplement that quality control personnel approve for reprocessing?*

§ 111.530 - *When must an investigation be conducted of your manufacturing processes and other batches?*

§ 111.535 - *Under this subpart N, what records must you make and keep?*

Subpart O--Product Complaints

§ 111.553 - *What are the requirements under this subpart O for written procedures?*

§ 111.560 - *What requirements apply to the review and investigation of a product complaint?*

§ 111.570 - *Under this subpart O, what records must you make and keep?*

Subpart P--Records and Recordkeeping

§ 111.605 - *What requirements apply to the records that you make and keep?*

§ 111.610 - *What records must be made available to FDA?*

From nothing to all of this?—Where do these dietary supplement companies even start. FDA is already in the process of inspecting dietary supplement companies for compliance with their new GMPS and has even started issuing Warning Letters.

This sounds like a great opportunity for consultants and employment for ex-pharma people. Not so fast. As with everything else new, it will only happen when dietary supplement company executives get their heads out of the sand and realize, after a bad inspection or Warning Letter that they don't understand what to do, or how to do it.

An example of a Warning Letter issued to a company in Texas is presented here for illustrative purposes. Please note the detail of this Warning Letter. It is very typical of what one would see in a drug Warning Letter. By the way, there are some food- terms used here as well, and for readers unfamiliar with food regulations, the term HACCP, cited in this Warning Letter, stands for Hazard Analysis by Critical Control Points. It is a system that is used in both food manufacturing and restaurants. Most food Warning Letters involves deficient HACCP or sanitation programs. OK, here's the dietary supplement Warning Letter, in its entirety, copied from FDA's web site (Public Information). The letter was issued by FDA on March 30, 2010.

WARNING LETTER

CERTIFIED   *MAIL*
RETURN RECEIPT REQUESTED

Dallas, Texas 75243

Dear Mr.:

On September 1 through September 18, 2009, the U.S. Food and Drug Administration (FDA) performed an inspection of your firm located at 9660 Dilworth Road, Dallas, Texas. Our investigator found a number of violations of 21 CFR Part 111, Current Good Manufacturing Practice (CGMP) in Manufacturing, Packaging, Labeling, or Holding Operations for Dietary Supplements.

The inspection revealed that your Herbalife Ready Herbal Aloe for Digestive Health Dietary Supplement and Herbalife Herbal Aloe Concentrate for Digestive Health Dietary Supplement, products manufactured in your facility, are adulterated within the meaning of Section 402(g)(1) of the Federal Food, Drug, and Cosmetic Act (the Act) in that the dietary supplements have been prepared, packed, or held under conditions that do not meet current good manufacturing practice regulations for dietary supplements. These observations were presented to you in an FDA-483 at the conclusion of our inspection on September 18, 2009.

The inspection revealed the following deficiencies:

*1. Your firm failed to conduct at least one appropriate test or examination to verify the identity of a dietary ingredient prior to its use, to comply with 21 CFR 111.75(a)(1)(i). Specifically, your firm uses aloe as an ingredient in your Herbalife Ready Herbal Aloe for Digestive Health Dietary Supplement (32 fl oz and 1 gallon sizes) and Herbalife Herbal Aloe Concentrate for Digestive Health Dietary Supplement, but your firm does not perform an appropriate identity test or examination on the aloe raw material. Although your firm performs **(b)(4)** and appearance testing for this material, such testing is not appropriate. As discussed with your staff, such testing would not indicate whether, for example, a dietary component was a mixture of aloe, thickeners, and/or other ingredients.*

*We acknowledge receipt of your October 12, 2009, response to the FDA 483; however, it does not adequately address your failure to conduct at least one appropriate test or examination to verify the identity of the aloe ingredient prior to its use. Your letter stated that you have ordered an aloe standard and that you would use the **(b)(4)** chromatography methodology accompanying the standard to verify the identity of aloe if you were able to successfully replicate that methodology. However, you did not specify how you intended to verify the identity of aloe used to manufacture your dietary supplements until December 18, 2009 (your anticipated correction date). Similarly, your letter did not specify the identity test or examination your firm would implement in the event that your firm could not successfully replicate the proposed identity methodology.*

2. Your firm failed to make and keep documentation for why meeting in-process specifications, in combination with meeting component specifications, helps ensure that the dietary supplement meets the specifications for identity, purity, strength, and composition; and for limits on those types of contamination that may adulterate or may lead to adulteration of the finished batch of the dietary supplement, to comply with 21 CFR 111.95(b)(3). Specifically, you have no documentation to explain the rationale behind the specifications that you have for raw materials(such as aloe, chamomile, water, citric acid, and preservatives) used in your dietary supplements and in-process samples (samples taken of product before packaging) of these dietary supplements. Additionally, you did not make and keep documentation demonstrating why the results of appropriate tests or examinations for the product specifications selected under 111.75(c)(1) ensure that your dietary supplements meets all product specifications, in accordance with 21 CFR 111.95(b)(4).

*Your October 12th response indicates your firm has begun implementation of a HACCP plan. While we acknowledge the evaluation of critical control points in the processing of dietary supplements can be useful, this response is inadequate because it did not indicate that your HACCP plan will document the rationale required under 21 CFR 111.95(b) (3) and (b)(4). Further, your letter states that you have created a new SOP titled "Development of a New **(b)(4)** Product," which was to be implemented by October 31, 2009. Your response states that the SOP will explain the rationale behind your manufacturing process, product specifications, and testing practice. However, your response is inadequate because you did not submit this SOP for our evaluation, and therefore, we cannot determine whether it meets the requirements of 21 CFR 111.95(b)(3) and (b)(4).*

*3. You did not follow your written procedure, "Approval/Rejection of Raw Materials and Packaging Components" for collecting representative samples of each unique shipment of components. Under 21 CFR 111.153, you must establish and follow written procedures for fulfilling the requirements of subpart G. This subpart includes the requirement that you collect representative samples of each unique lot of components (21 CFR 111.155(c)(1)). Specifically, you did not follow your written procedures stating that you will sample the **(b)(4)** of the number* *of containers in a shipment. Our investigator observed that only one box of potassium sorbate had been opened for sampling out of a shipment of **(b)(4)** boxes. Also, only one bag of trisodium citrate dihydrate had been opened for sampling out of a shipment of **(b)(4)** bags.*

*Your October 12th response indicated that your firm's SOP "Approval/ Rejection of Raw Materials and Packaging Components" was revised to better define "container." Your response states that "container" is now defined as a **(b)(4)** and, with this change, multiple cases will be sampled across a single manufacturer's lot of raw material or packaging components. The revised SOP was to be implemented by November 20, 2009. Your response does not adequately address this observation because it does not provide assurance that your staff has been trained to follow your written procedures for collecting representative samples.*

4. Your quality control program is not adequate. For example:

a. Your quality control operations did not include periodic review of all records for calibration of instruments and controls, as required by 21 CFR 111.117(b). Specifically, your firm does not periodically review calibration records for production equipment, including scales and water meters used to measure dietary supplement ingredients.

Your response letter indicates SOP 1590, "Quality Review of Equipment/Instrument Calibrations" was implemented on October 7, 2009, and that QC will review records for all equipment requiring calibration through the plant. However, your response did not include a copy of the new SOP or evidence of implementation. We will address the sufficiency of this correction during the next inspection.

*b. Your master manufacturing record does not include written instructions for manual operations that include one person verifying the addition of a component, as required by 21 CFR 111.210(h) (3)(ii)(B). Specifically, you have one employee working in the food compounding area **(b)(4)**. This employee adds components of your dietary supplements without a second employee verifying the addition. According to management, a **(b)(4)** employee checks the next day to ensure that the **(b)(4)** employee has completed the* *required paperwork, and signs off on the paperwork to indicate that he has done so. However, your master manufacturing record does not include instructions that the addition of components by one employee must be verified by another employee.*

Your response indicates that all dietary supplement compounding activities were moved to (b)(4) and your firm is currently evaluating resources to support future (b)(4). This response is not adequate because it does not indicate that you have revised your master manufacturing record to include a second employee verifying the addition of a component by another employee. We will address the sufficiency of this correction during the next inspection.

c. Your firm failed to include documentation, at the time of performance, in the batch production record that quality control personnel approved and released, or rejected, the packaged and labeled dietary supplement, including any repackaged or relabeled dietary supplement, to comply with 21 CFR 111.260(1)(4). Specifically, our investigator observed that quality control personnel did not document approval and release, or rejection, of the finished product in the batch production record. Although the quality assurance forms in your batch records document review of appropriate records, they do not document release of finished product.

Your response letter indicates that forms QA041 and QA042 will be revised to clearly state: "Batch Released by Quality Assurance:_____," the line indicating signature and date. Your letter specifies that corrections were to be completed by October 31, 2009. This response is inadequate because it does not explain that your personnel have been trained to use these revised forms to document release or rejection of a dietary supplement at the time of performance. We will address the sufficiency of this correction during the next inspection.

5. Your master manufacturing record did not include a statement of the theoretical yield of a manufactured dietary supplement expected at each point, step, or stage of the manufacturing process where control is needed to ensure the quality of the dietary supplement, and the expected yield when you finish manufacturing the dietary supplement, to comply with 21 CFR 111.210(f).

Your response indicates that your batch production records will be revised to include a section to record bulk yields, and a bulk yield specification will be added to the in-process release specification section of the batch production records. This response is inadequate because it addresses changes you intend to make to your batch production records, rather than your master manufacturing records.

6. Your batch production records did not include a statement of the percentage of theoretical yield at appropriate phases of processing in accordance with 21 CFR 111.260(f).

Your response indicates revisions will be made to all batch production records for dietary supplements to include a section for recording bulk yields. Your response states, in addition, that a bulk yield specification will be added to the in-process release specification section of the batch production records, and that your firm will also revise the Job Completion Report to include a statement of the percentage of theoretical yield at appropriate phases of processing. However, this response is inadequate because you have not provided a copy of these revisions. We will address the sufficiency of these corrections during the next inspection.

7. The written instructions in your master manufacturing records did not include corrective action plans to use when a specification is not met, in accordance with 21 CFR 111.210(h)(5).

Your letter indicates the statement, "If the above standard specifications are not met, a product investigation will be initiated to determine the root cause," will be added to the Standard Specifications section of the batch production record. This response is inadequate because it indicates that you intend to revise your batch production records, rather than your master manufacturing records.

This letter is not an all-inclusive list of violations at your facility. It is your responsibility to ensure that your establishment and the products you market comply with the Act and its implementing regulations.

Failure to promptly correct the violations specified above may result in enforcement action without further notice. Enforcement action may include seizure of violative products and/or injunction against the manufacturers and distributors of violative products.

Please advise this office in writing within 15 days from your receipt of this letter of the specific steps you have taken to correct the violations noted above and to ensure that similar violations do not occur. Your response should include any documentation necessary to show that correction has been achieved. If you cannot complete all corrections before you respond, state the reason for the delay and the date by which you will complete the corrections.

Please send your reply to the Food and Drug Administration, Attention: Sherrie L. Krolczyk, Compliance Officer, at the above letterhead address. If you have any questions regarding any issue in this letter, please contact Sherrie L. Krolczyk at (214) 253-5312.

Sincerely,

Reynaldo R. Rodriguez, Jr.
Dallas District Director

Holy cow, what a shellacking and we are sure to see many more like this. This looks like a typical drug Warning Letter, maybe worse. Problem is, dietary supplement companies aren't used to this sort of thing and probably don't know what to do about it. I personally contacted this firm, offering my assistance to help them remediate the Warning Letter and return the company to a state of acceptable compliance. I was told that their GMPs are just fine. For Pete's sake, how can anyone who has just received such a Warning Letter possibly believe that their GMP compliance is acceptable.

The above is just one example. As FDA continues to inspect dietary supplement manufacturers and enforce the new GMPs, we will surely see more of the same. Growing pains will take some time, but at least as consumers, we are bound to be better off than before when it comes to reliability, consistency and safety of dietary supplements that are sold in the United States.

Over time, after many FDA inspections, data will become available through inspection reports, Warning Letters and recalls that will allow us to better decide from which companies we want to purchase our dietary supplements.

Finally, keep in mind that many of the problems discussed for OTC generic drugs such as use of questionable ingredients and shoddy manufacturing practices often also apply to the nutritional supplement industry.

CHAPTER FOUR

REAL GENERIC STORIES
—NILSEN'S BELIEVE IT OR NOT

No discussion of the generic world, particularly the generic OTC world would be complete without relating some wild and sometimes amusing tales of experiences and observations that could make one gasp in total disbelief. The six-pack of stories told in this chapter are a retelling of actual personal experiences at actual drug and dietary supplement companies, that further justify my personal preference for brand name over generic OTC drugs. This time for the sake of mercy and avoidance of embarrassment, company names are withheld.

As you read these, keep in mind that anyone can start up a generic OTC company in their basement or garage so long as they manufacture under GMPs. However, many small operators don't even know what GMPs are and just blindly jump into the drug manufacturing business. It will probably be a good year or more until they get their first FDA inspection, but in the meanwhile, products are going out the door. Wouldn't it make more sense to have an inspection <u>before</u> a company is allowed to distribute drug products?

Story #1 (Southeast New Jersey)

I did an audit of a plant that made active drug ingredients (APIs). This was a large, well-known player in the industry. The warehouse doors had large holes in them allowing rodents and other pests to run wild. Label control was no good and many lab instruments were not calibrated, plus, observations from previous FDA inspections were never corrected. The head of quality had been aware of these things for months. Management did not respond to any of this with any sense of urgency, suggesting that they really don't care. FDA will care during their next inspection. Unfortunately, many companies fit this profile of talking a good GMP show, but not backing it up with action.

Story #2 (New York State)

This one is classic and of gargantuan proportions. Were it not for personal experience, this could have classified as science fiction. There was a large generic company that employed about forty five analytical chemists. These are chemists that do drug testing. For some reason about half of the work done always had to be repeated because of one problem or another, which totally destroyed productivity and efficiency. Now if a lab test gives an out of specification results, the result should be investigated to see if it is explainable and to see if the original bad result can be legitimately discarded and replaced by new passing results. There is a process for doing this that is clearly defined in current FDA guidance documents. However, back in 1990 when this was going on, no clear guidance existed.

At this company, if a test result failed, the test was repeated by the original chemist, then by other chemists and then on re-samples until a passing result was obtained. In other words, product was tested into compliance, without any scientifically sound justification for accepting a passing result in lieu of a failing one. It was anybody's guess if a product released for sale was actually good or not. Boy, that's reassuring. As a Six Sigma Master Black Belt, I am adamant about building quality into a product by design. In other words, quality is already there, and testing merely confirms it. The chemist doing the testing is in a sense acting as a coroner, if the batch is no good, it is pronounced dead. No amount of testing or retesting will impart quality that is not already there.

Well, the first step was to measure the competence of the chemists. Was product quality really bad, or were the lab chemist simply incapable of generating reliable test results. A simple lab performance test was designed that would clearly demonstrate whether or not chemists possessed the basic technique skills necessary to perform acceptable laboratory testing work. It consisted of five basic operations, performed sequentially. Any competent analytical chemist would be expected to execute the five steps flawlessly and without incident.

So, the test was administered to all forty five chemists. Guess what percentage of chemists was able to pass the test, i.e., execute all five steps properly? The answer is zero. Not one chemist could get through this exercise without making major errors. The outcome was quite startling, have never seen anything like it actually, and when the results were presented to management, there response was basically—bullshit, we can't accept the fact that all forty five chemists are fundamentally incompetent. The company president even remarked that his chemists were the industry's finest. God help us at the time if that was true.

Was the test too hard or unfair, well, the same test was given to 120 chemists at a major brand name company (Hoffman-LaRoche), and guess what, every single chemist passed with flying colors and no errors. The difference, in my mind, was a combination of poor training, language skills, quality of supervision and hiring practices at the generic firm.

The company had many problems, not only in laboratory testing but in manufacturing as well. How could anything produced by this company at that point in time be trusted? By the way, this is same company that during an FDA inspection, proved beyond the shadow of a doubt that a batch or product was destroyed five months before it was manufactured, remember?

Story #3 (Northern New Jersey)

This one we touched upon in an earlier chapter, but is presented here in greater detail for everyone's amusement.—talk about science fiction! As drug companies go, this one was at the low end of the spectrum; the absolute bottom of the barrel. As mentioned earlier, the building leaked like a sieve—on rainy days it rained indoors, dogs were allowed to frolic through the facility, microbiological contamination was rampant and employees who spoke English were as rare as hen's teeth. In addition, laboratory data was forged and product quality was suspect at best. Their products consisted mainly of creams and ointments, some antibiotic in nature, packaged in tubes and single-dose foil packs. Their definition of GMP was Generate More Profit. Their products were clearly not fit for sale to consumers.

During a tough FDA inspection, where they were getting hammered, the owners called me in as a consultant to help get them out from under the mess they were in. A remediation plan was developed that bought them a few months' time, but to no avail. A few weeks after the inspection ended, a recall had to be initiated because a product that was shipped to a nursing home was found to contain dangerous gram-negative bacteria. One morning, about a week or so after the recall, I came into the plant about 7:30 AM and got this weird feeling that today is the day something is going to happen. Sure enough, about half an hour later, four guys built like professional wrestlers march into the building with guns and badges, identify themselves and U.S. Marshalls and proceed to execute an arrest warrant. All goods were seized and all employees were sent home. It was game over for that company, who was never again allowed to make or distribute drug products in the United States. By the way, this outfit is still in business selling cosmetics. During the U.S. Marshall's visit, the building was surrounded by news media folks. I hid in the rodent-infested basement to avoid being seen.

Story #4 (South Carolina)

A guy in South Carolina who was in the textile business, one day decided to start a drug company. He set up shop (remember anyone can start up and get going in their garage or basement) and started cranking out drug products. His company made cough and cold products that were generic imitations of brand name products. As a contract laboratory owner at the time, I contracted with him to do the lab testing on all his products. Well one product after another came out great, just as good as the brand product.

Were these products really that good? Well, to make a long story short, something was fishy, and after reviewing the lab data and subsequent conversations with FDA's criminal investigations branch, it was discovered that the samples sent to us for testing were actually the brand product that was put into their bottles, so that the analysis would always come out good and they could ship their crap to market. One example was a product called Nite Time, which is a generic OTC version of the brand drug Nyquil®. Well, the company was putting Nyquil® in bottles labeled with their product Nite Time. Of course it tested good, Nyquil® is a great product that consistently meets specifications.

Do you think that this is the only generic OTC-company that was doing this sort of thing? Still interested in saving a few bucks?

Story #5 (Southeast Pennsylvania)

A small family-owned pharmaceutical firm with limited financial resources that talked a good quality show, unless of course it costs too much, was making products containing glycerin. Remember our discussion about glycerin and antifreeze? By the way, this outfit bought a lot of ingredients from China and India.

They tested their glycerin on a piece of laboratory equipment that had no provision for making sure that data generated was secure and could not be altered. Under GMPs, data from such an instrument cannot be used to make decisions about releasing raw materials or products to market. Yet, they released and approved glycerin and other raw materials for use that were tested on that instrument, a clear violation of GMPs. But why? Isn't there anything that could have been done? Sure thing— just upgrade the software that controls the instrument to make it GMP-complaint. The upgrade was refused because of price. It was decided to continue using this instrument to test glycerin and other raw materials, rather than spend a lousy six thousand dollars for an upgrade. With this company, despite potential risk to consumers, quality comes first unless it is too expensive. There were other situations as well where GMPS were bypassed to get product out the door. The problem was resolved when a former senior employee contacted FDA and blew the whistle on the company, triggering an inspection.

Story #6 (Central Pennsylvania)

A chemical company that made additives had an interesting habit of always finding a way to pass a lot of chemicals regardless of the quality, unless the stuff was so off the wall that nobody would buy it. They had about two million dollars' worth of that crap lying around waiting to be reworked or discarded.

This company used to change the particle size of materials by putting it through what was called a beading tower. These beading towers contained mercury-well thermometers, a no-no for towers in which food or other consumable products are made. Well guess what? A mercury-well thermometer in a food-grade tower broke resulting in product contaminated with mercury. The problem was not discovered until a fair amount of product wound up on the market.

The quality control manager demanded a product recall. The plant manager refused, because he was also committed to quality so long as it did not interfere with profit or looking good to his superiors. The quality control manager threatened to call FDA if the product wasn't voluntarily recalled, and was fired for his trouble. Stuck in central Pennsylvania, it took me five months to find another job.

These stories are not uncommon, the point being that there are a lot of companies that don't or can't take quality and compliance seriously. And, it is often the small mom and pop drug companies that fall into this category. There are many aspects to drug product manufacturing starting with making the ingredients in a chemical plant followed by the finished product drug manufacturer performing a multitude of operations such as pharmacy dispensing, blending, granulation, tableting, encapsulation, grinding, drying, packaging and labeling to name a few. All of these activities should be performed under strict GMPs and with an unwavering upper management commitment to quality and compliance.

Consider all of this when purchasing OTC drug products. Whether it's a pain killer, antihistamine, decongestant, combination cold product or any other common remedy, I strongly recommend sticking with the brand if possible. I'll take my Nyquil®, Bayer® Aspirin, Robitussin®, Zyrtec®, Benadryl® and other brand dugs any day of the week over their generic counterparts. I'm just not in the mood to get poisoned or injured by products contaminated with antifreeze, melamine, glass and metal particles or harmful bacteria.

Don't get me wrong. Many generics OTC drugs are just fine, however, since you can't always be sure of the manufacturer, proceed with caution.

Some OTC products mention the manufacturer's name on their label. In these cases you can check out the manufacturer for yourself. Chapter 6, "Self Defense" shows you how.

CHAPTER FIVE

ACTIVE PHARMACEUTICAL INGREDIENTS

No view of the pharmaceutical industry would be complete without a discussion of the active ingredients used in drug products—what they are, how they are made and how does FDA protect consumers from harm? This short chapter will introduce you to the very important world of active pharmaceutical ingredients.

Active pharmaceutical ingredients, better known as APIs, are chemicals that are made in chemical plants. There are many different kinds of chemicals that are used in a variety of applications such as the manufacture of pesticides, plastics, industrial products and many others. APIs are chemicals that have a therapeutic effect, i.e., they act on the body in a therapeutic way. APIs can be decongestants, cough suppressants, antihistamines, pain killers or antacids for example. APIs are used in drug products to treat a myriad of health problems ranging from heart disease and cancer to more rare and exotic diseases. Keep in mind though that APIs are chemicals and as such, require careful evaluation as to benefits versus safety and side effects. Remember the earlier discussion of how a new drug gets approved? Well, every new API that comes along goes through that long and expensive process to be sure that it is both safe and effective.

Some APIs are relatively non-toxic and can be easily manufactured and handled with minimal precautions, while others are highly potent compounds that must be made and handled in special isolators. Some are so potent, usually the anti-cancer drugs, that an amount too small to see with the human eye, micrograms, can be toxic. One example is a drug called carmustine, a very simple mustard gas-related molecule that is used to treat various cancers, including brain tumors. It has a potency rating of four (highest you can go on the Safebridge® potency scale) and is unbelievably toxic. The bottom line is always whether or not the benefits outweigh the risks. Drugs like carmustine kill cancer, but they can also kill you. Please talk to your doctor about the benefits and risks of any drug that's prescribed for you.

So, there are dangers associated with APIs as well as benefits. Aside from potency, why? Well, it has to do with how APIs are made. As mentioned, APIs are chemicals that are made in chemical plants, and even though these chemical plants are FDA regulated, they are still chemical plants. APIs are made in typical fashion by reacting different chemicals together through processes that may include heating, cooling, filtering, distillation, centrifuging or drying, to name a few. The chemicals used to make an API are its raw materials that can themselves be dangerous. Just like an API is a raw material in a drug product, chemicals are the raw material for the API. Even though the API manufacturing process will usually include purification steps, there can still be some left over impurities from the manufacturing process that remain in the API. Don't get too excited, this is normal. The real question is how many impurities, how much of each, and what is their potency and/or therapeutic effect, and how are the quantities of each impurity controlled so they stay within safe limits?

There two basic types of impurities; the first is an impurity that has no therapeutic effect. In other words, it doesn't act like a drug. The other is an impurity that does act like a drug, also known as a related substance. These need to be extra-carefully controlled in order that a prescribed dose of drug product doesn't artificially boost the active ingredient effect due to the presence of related substances.

OK, here's where the FDA steps in. The GMPs for APIs are contained in a guidance put out by the International Conference on Harmonisation, specifically ICH Q7, " Good Manufacturing

Practice Guidance for Active Pharmaceutical Ingredients". FDA inspects API manufacturers for compliance with this guidance (Q7). ICH Q7 spells out requirements for "Quality Management"," Personnel, Buildings and Facilities", "Process Equipment"," Documentation and Records"," Materials Management", "Production and In-Process Controls", "Packaging and Identification Labeling of APIs and Intermediates"," Laboratory Controls", "Validation", "Change Control", "Rejection and Re-Use of Materials", "Complaints and Recalls", "Contract Manufacturers (Including Laboratories)", "Agents, Brokers, Traders, Distributors, Repackers and Relabellers", and "Specific Guidance for APIs Manufactured by Cell Culture/Fermentation".

There are many areas of similarly between drug product regulation and API regulation, but also, there are many facets of the regulations that are directed specifically towards API production. Keep in mind that because of the nature of chemical reactions, there are very strict safety and handling considerations. APIs have much tighter specifications than drug products. Not only do they have to be very pure, they must contain very low levels of impurities. For me though, the biggest problem with API regulation is where APIs come from.

Drug product manufacturers are required by GMPs to qualify their suppliers, who are API manufacturers, which often involve actual site visits to the supplier's facility. Well if the API supplier is in the United States, no big deal. Visit them every two years or so to audit them for compliance with Q7. But wait a minute, what about those suppliers, and there are many, who are located in places like China and India?

Even big companies do not like spending money on trips to Asia, but many small companies simply can't afford it or don't want to spend the money. But guess what? It's the small companies, the small generic companies in particular, who buy these APIs from places like China and India. Even FDA has trouble with foreign inspections due to manpower and language issues. Fortunately, FDA has set up resident posts in many foreign countries with native-speaking investigators.

But for the small generic OTC manufacturer, who is always looking for bargains, as we say in New York," forget about it". Even if one were to audit a Chinese API factory for example, they would need a translator which makes auditing very difficult. A colleague and good friend of mine, who has spent a lot of time in China, assures me that many Chinese drug and API companies lie like rugs though their translators to get a favorable audit result. Unless one brings their own translator, or better yet an auditor who is a native language speaker, it just isn't possible to get an accurate assessment of the company's compliance status.

There are many API factories in China, many of whom are of questionable repute. It's the smaller generic OTC companies who tend to buy Chinese or Indian APIs because of price, and it is the smaller generic OTC companies that generally don't conduct on-site audits of foreign companies. Check out results of this inspection:

DEPARTMENT OF HEALTH AND HUMAN SERVICES	
FOOD AND DRUG ADMINISTRATION	
DISTRICT OFFICE ADDRESS AND PHONE NUMBER International Compliance Team, DMPQ/OC/CDER, FDA White Oak Building 51, 4th FLoor 10903 New Hampshire Avenue Silver Spring, MD 20993 USA **[Handwritten #1: adding the phone number "(301) 827-8942"]**	DATE(S) OF INSPECTION Feb 20, 21, 22, 25 & 26, 2008
	DATE(S) OF INSPECTION Feb 20, 21, 22, 25 & 26, 2008
NAME AND TITLE OF INDIVIDUAL TO WHOM REPORT IS ISSUED **TO:** Mr. Yan Wang, General Manager	
FIRM NAME Changzhou SPL Company, Ltd.	STREET ADDRESS 3 Changhong West Road
CITY, STATE AND ZIP CODE Wujing, Changzhou City, Jiangsu Province, China	TYPE OF ESTABLISHMENT INSPECTED API (animal origin) Manufacturer

THIS DOCUMENT LISTS OBSERVATIONS MADE BY THE FDA REPRESENTATIVE(S) DURING THE INSPECTION OF YOUR FACILITY. THEY ARE INSPECTIONAL OBSERVATIONS, AND DO NOT REPRESENT A FINAL AGENCY DETERMINATION REGARDING YOUR COMPLIANCE. IF YOU HAVE AN OBJECTION REGARDING AN OBSERVATION, OR HAVE IMPLEMENTED. OR PLAN TO IMPLEMENT. CORRECTIVE ACTION IN RESPONSE TO AN OBSERVATION. YOU MAY DISCUSS THE OBJECTION OR ACTION WITH THE FDA REPRESENTATIVE(S) DURING THE INSPECTION OR SUBMIT THIS INFORMATION TO FDA AT THE ADDRESS ABOVE. IF YOU HAVE ANY QUESTIONS, PLEASE CONTACT FDA AT THE PHONE NUMBER AND ADDRESS ABOVE.

DURING AN INSPECTION OF YOUR FIRM (I) (WE) OBSERVED:

1. There have been no critical processing steps identified for the Heparin Sodium USP **[Redacted]** process, and, the repeated and efficient removal of impurities, such as proteins, nucleotides, virus, endotoxin, bacteria and heavy metals at the appropriate, specified, process steps has not been evaluated. There was no report for annual **[Redacted]** test results available.

   The improvements offered by removal of a raw material **[Redacted]** test @ **[Redacted]** a batch size increase, an added **[Redacted]** step, a change in **[Redacted]** for the **[Redacted]** step and **[Redacted]** and parameter changes, approved in a 1/05 process validation report for Heparin Sodium USP, were not demonstrated.

2. There has been no impurity profile established for Heparin Sodium USP and no evaluation for degradants during stability program testing.

3. The manufacturing instructions for Heparin Sodium USP are incomplete in that they do not include a description of manual manipulations of the **[Redacted]** during processing steps, they do not include the actual, manually entered **[Redacted]** set temperatures and times and, operator observations such as level measurements, used in calculations, during the **[Redacted]** step are not recorded.

4. There has been no test method verification performed for the reported USP test methods, Nitrogen Determination, Protein and Total Aerobic Microbial Count, employed in testing of Heparin Sodium USP and Heparin Crude materials, to show that the methods are suitable under actual conditions of use. In addition, there is no routine test for [Redacted] residue amount at the time of release.

5. Investigations into failed lots and out of trend lots were approved as complete, but did not identify a cause for the problem. For example,

   Heparin Sodium USP batch [Redacted] failed the Nitrogen Determination test and was reprocessed to make [Redacted] without finding the reason for the slightly high, OOS Nitrogen result.

   Investigations into [Handwritten #2: cross out a word, added "OOT"] of customer [Redacted] specification @[Redacted] for Heparin Sodium USP lots [Handwritten #3: cross out word(s)] [Redacted] and [Handwritten #4: cross out word.] were performed without knowing what the failed test measurement actually represented.

   [Redacted][Handwritten #5: added "and the failure of lot"] [Redacted]

   Investigations into ROI out of trend results for Heparin Sodium USP lots [Redacted] identified both results inappropriately as outliers.

6. Heparin Crude lots [Redacted] received 8/06 from vendor [Handwritten #6: cross out word(s)] [Redacted] that included material from an unacceptable workshop vendor were used in Heparin Sodium USP [Redacted] marketed to the USA. In addition, prior to 3/06 there are no [Redacted] records from vendor [Redacted] showing the source for their crude materials.

7. The inside surface of large, "cleaned" **[Redacted]** tanks used in the final **[Redacted]** step, after both **[Redacted]** were very scratched, with unidentified material adhering to the insides and, the inverted handles held liquid, which spilled to the bottom of the tank when it was uprighted. There was no written procedure showing that the tanks were dedicated to a particular process step. There was no data collected to verify marker and tape volume markings on the outside of the tanks and, the cleaning method was not validated. It was noted that equipment cleaning tags were made of paper and taped to the piece of equipment unprotected from liquids used in the processing room environments.

8. Raw material inventory records were incomplete in that samples removed from the containers and the status and amount of materials returned from use by the production processing department were not recorded. For **[Redacted]** stored in a freezer, the amount, condition and date of return was not recorded.

9. Control of material flow in the processing area was inadequate in that waste **[Redacted]** was carted through a door to the outside in the processing area and not provided for by the material flow written procedure.

10. The outer foil bags containing Heparin Sodium USP lot **[Redacted]** manufactured and held since 5/25/07, are not labeled. The drum lid showed the only indications of the lot number.

11. There is no report or data to show that leachables for the **[Redacted]** bags used to hold Heparin Sodium USP lot, have been evaluated.

SEE REVERSE OF THIS PAGE	EMPLOYEE(S) SIGNATURE	EMPLOYEE(S) NAME AND TITLE (Print or Type)	DATE ISSUED
	[Signed] Regina T. Brown, Investigator Zi-Qiang Gu, Chemist	Regina T. Brown, Investigator Zi-Qiang Gu, Chemist	02/26/2008

So there you have it; companies using APIs in drug products that come from places like China. What companies?—generic OTC manufacturers. Once again, the buyer should beware. India also has API quality issues, but at least there, English is widely spoken.

On final topic—inactive ingredients, known as excipients, are also major ingredients of any drug product. Aside from the API, which is the active ingredient, every drug product you buy contains a number of excipients. Tablets for example would contain not only the API but other chemicals such as binders that help tablets stick together, disintegrants that allow a tablet to come apart in your stomach, lubricants and flow enhancers so blends will flow smoothly and not stick to the tablet press when being formed into tablets. Tablets might also contain a color or coating. Liquid products such as cough syrups could contain API plus purified water, sweeteners, flavors, colors, preservatives and thickeners for example. In the case of liquids, careful control must be exercised to prevent microbiological contamination, which can come from excipients or water.

Excipients are also subject to regulatory standards, specifically, they have to meet certain specifications set forth in standard reference books such as the National Formulary, which is part of the USP. Safety of excipients is coming under more careful review as well. What about purity and impurities? Finally, it should be noted that with excipients, drug companies generally accept a manufacturer's certificate of analysis and don't actually test the material themselves—they trust the supplier that the material is OK. Considering where some of this stuff could be coming from, maybe blindly trusting a supplier might not be such a great idea.

Once again, when it comes to OTC products, you often don't know who made the product or where their ingredients came from. No thanks, I'll take the brand name product any day.

CHAPTER SIX

SELF DEFENSE

These poor bastards are on their way home after making an uninformed purchase of some generic OTC drugs. Are you or your family in the same boat?

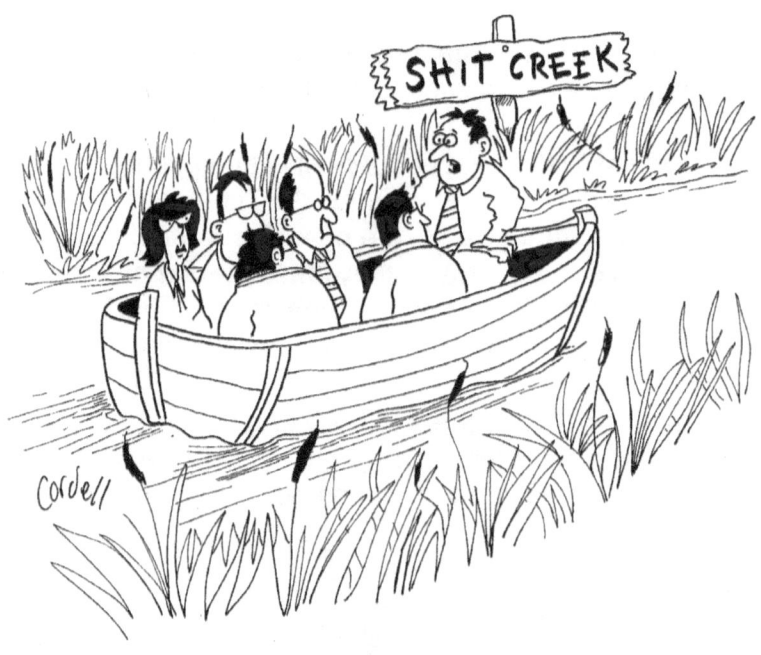

"What! *Nobody* thought to bring a paddle?"

OK, how do you protect yourself against buying or using drugs made or distributed by unreliable companies; you know, the ones who cut corners on quality, use cheap, unreliable ingredients or are always in trouble with FDA. This chapter is designed to present useful and practical means of self-defense for the drug-consuming public.

The best self -defense tool is the FDA website. We will go through a step by step process of browsing the site, showing you how to access all the information needed to be a smarter, more fully informed consumer. Let's log onto www.fda.gov. Once you log on and the home page comes up, you can see that there is tons of neat stuff to look at. *NOTE: Screen shots are from the time of this writing. Actual screen shot content, the FDA home page in particular, changes frequently. However, once you find and click on either Warning Letters of Enforcement Reports, the procedures described herein will work no matter when they are used and you will still be able to access the actual examples used in this chapter.*

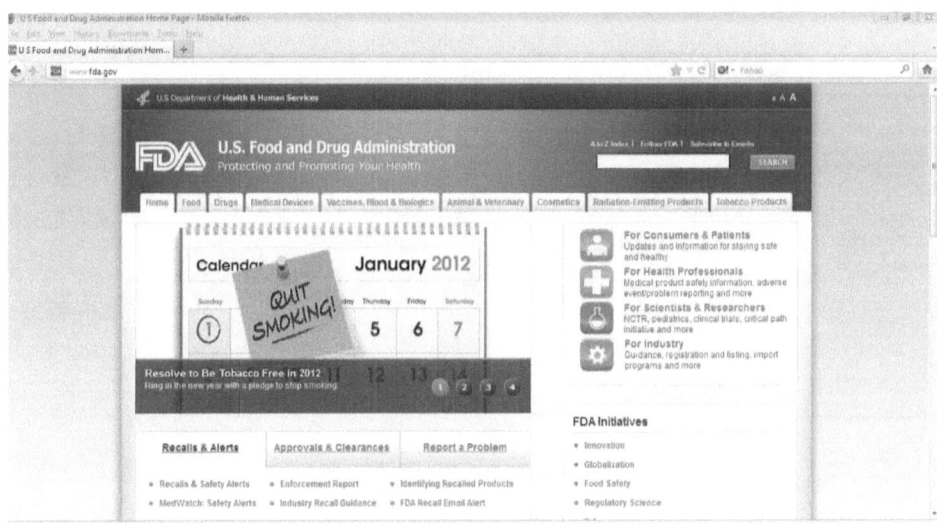

Figure 1

We talked quite extensively about Warning Letters, now we'll look at how to find them yourselves. Scroll-down the home page until you get to the bottom as shown in Figure 2.

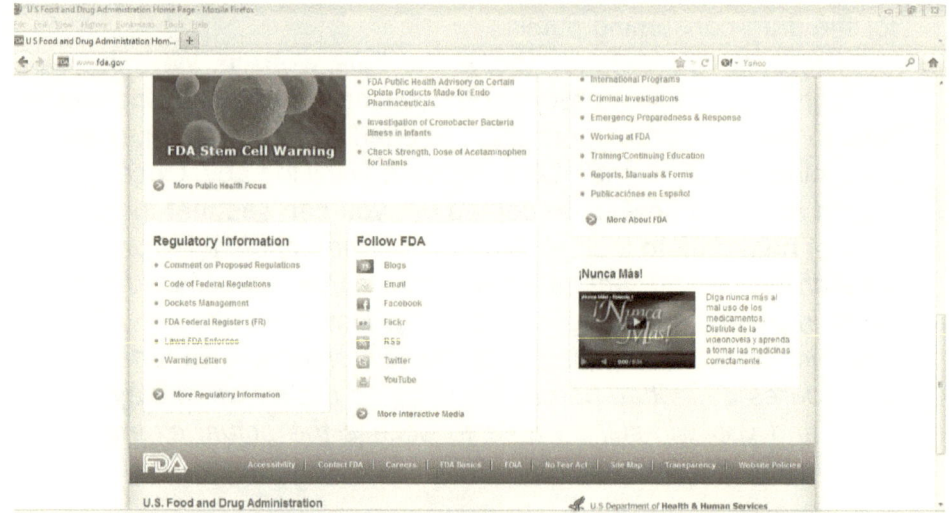

Figure 2

Under **Regulatory Information**, click on "**Warning Letters**" and a new screen appears, that allows one to browse warning letters a number of different ways such as by most recent, by date, by company and more.

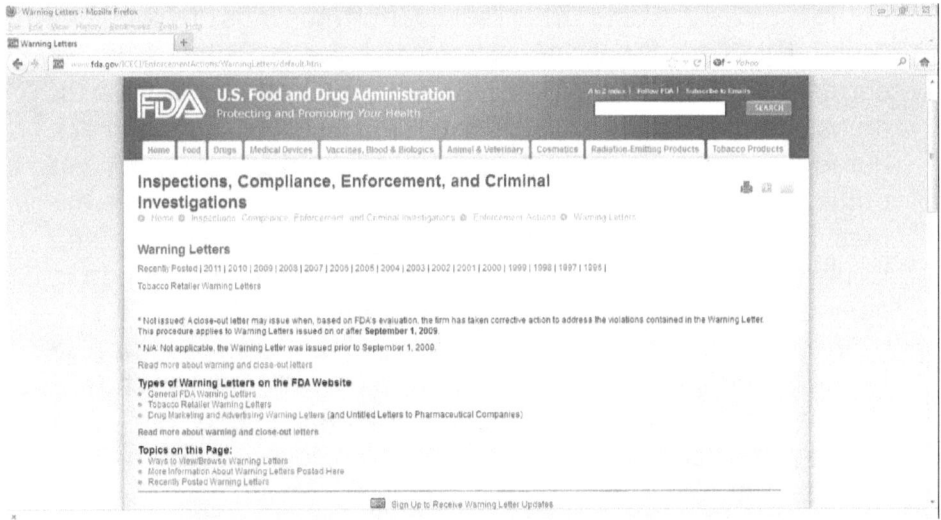

Figure 3

On this screen, click on "**Recently Posted Warning Letters**".

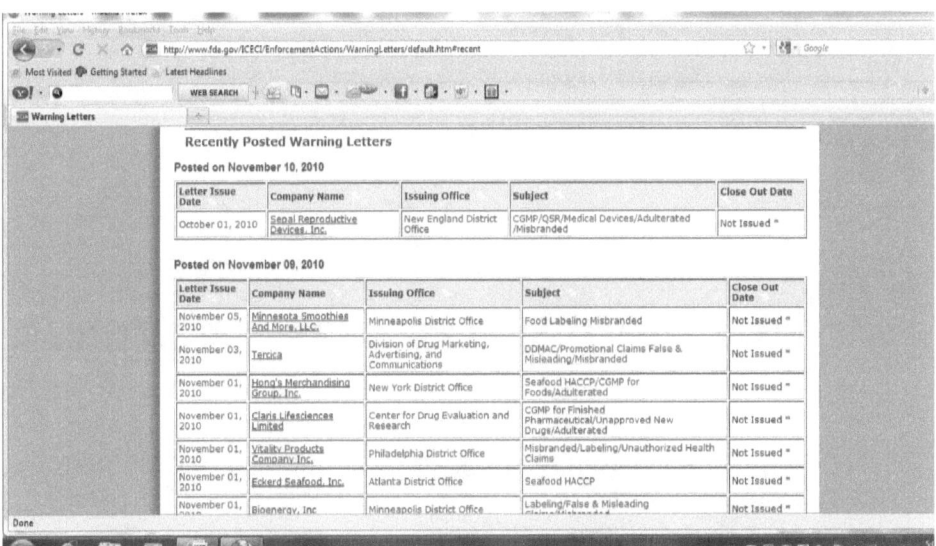

Figure 4

The above Warning Letter listing is from postings of November 9 and 10, 2010. What you will actually see in Figure 4, is the current listing for today's date. It includes Warning Letters for drugs, foods and medical devices, which allow one to check out food companies and medical device manufactures; not just drugs. This report only has one drug Warning Letter. To see the most recent Warning Letters, simply log onto FDAs website and follow the steps outlined above. A new Warning Letter report is generally published on Tuesday afternoons.

Now, let's search for other Warning Letters. Referring to Figure 3, under the banner **Warning Letters**, one can choose a recently posted Warning Letters plus Warning Letters for years ranging from current back to1996 (at the time of this writing). Let's try one. Click on **2009**.

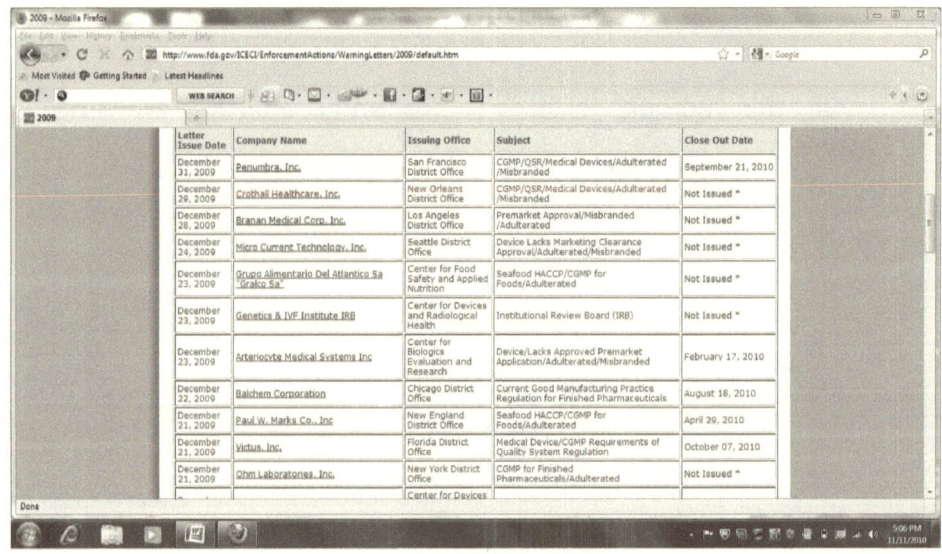

Figure 5

Every Warning Letter for the year 2009 is listed. To go through the list, simply scroll down. At the bottom of the page, click **[next]** to view the next page or **[previous]** to view a previous page.

This next one is very useful for the drug-consuming public. Suppose you purchased a drug product and would like to look at that company's Warning Letter history. Once again, referring to Figure 3, click on **"Ways to View/Browse Warning Letters"**.

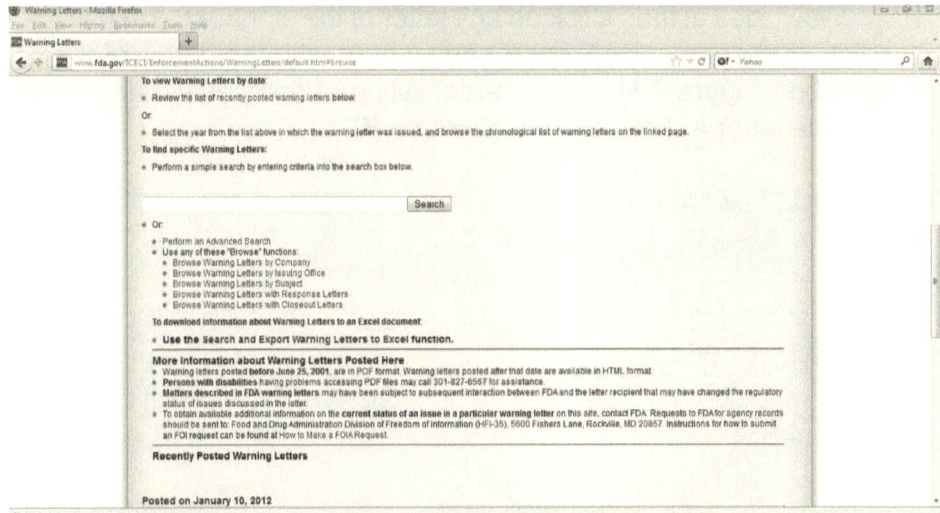

Figure 6

Now, looking at the left-hand side of the page shown in Figure 6, click on **"Browse Warning Letters by Company"**.

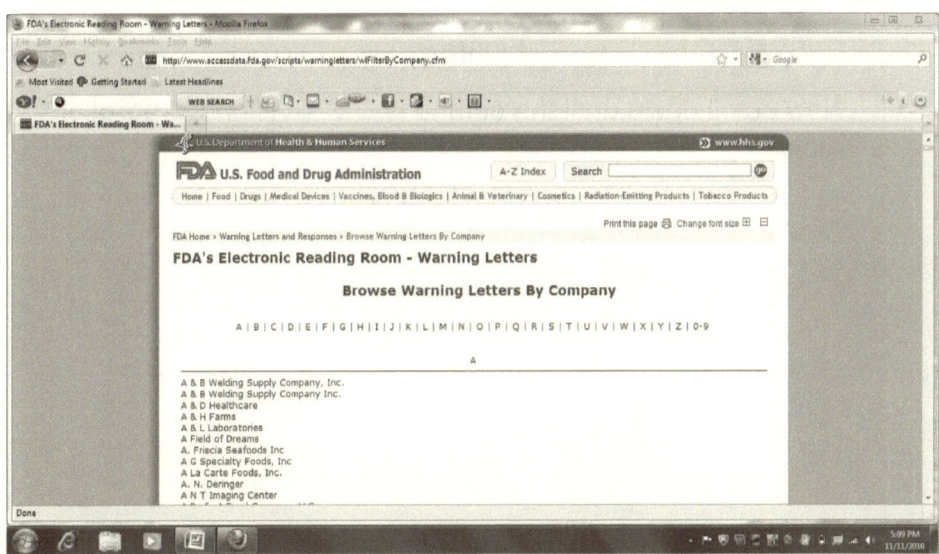

Figure 7

Wow, look at that. Click on any letter of the alphabet to display a listing of companies whose names start with that letter of the alphabet. Figure 7 shows a partial listing of companies starting with the letter A. Let's try one. Click on |C|.

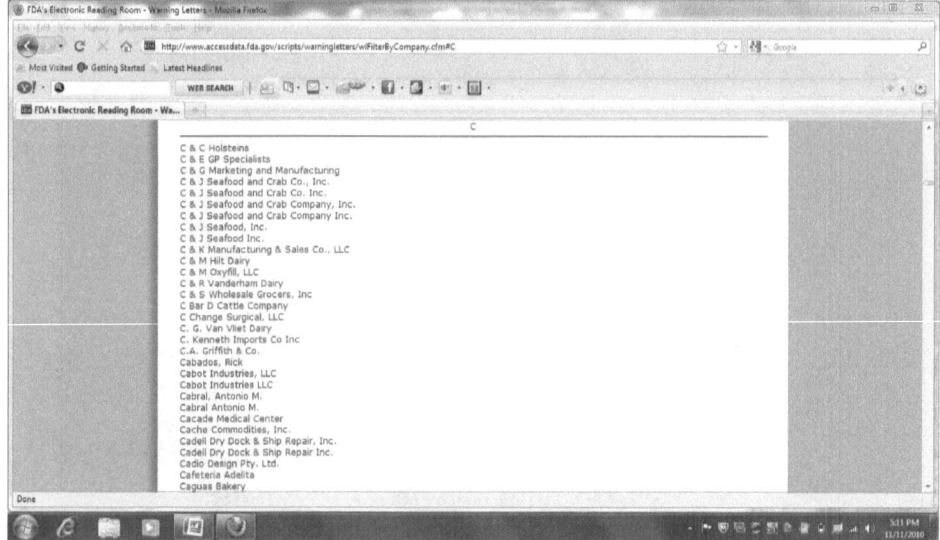

Figure 8

Now scroll down until the company CIBA-Vision Corporation is visible.

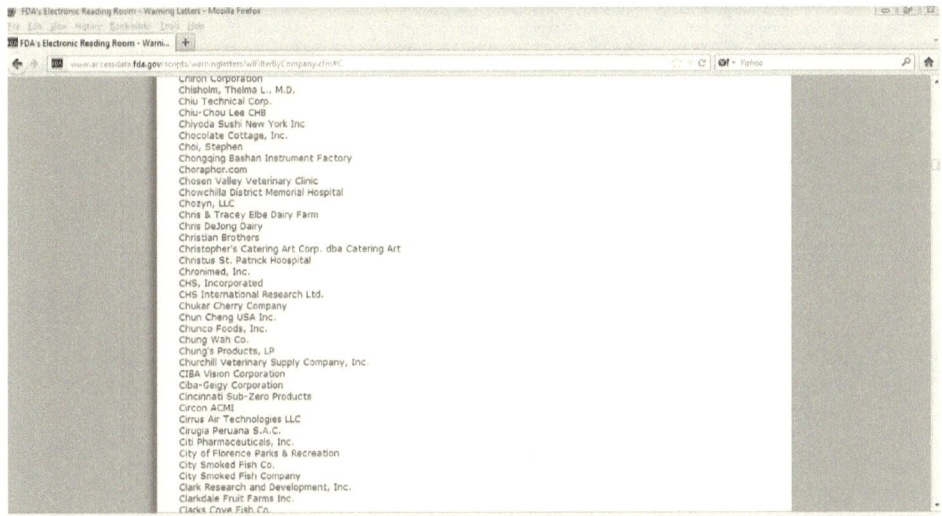

Figure 9

Click on CIBA-Vision Corporation. Then, referring to Figure 10, click on CIBA-Vision Corporation. The entire Warning Letter is displayed for your reading pleasure. As mentioned in an earlier chapter, note the similarity in Warning Letters from company to company.

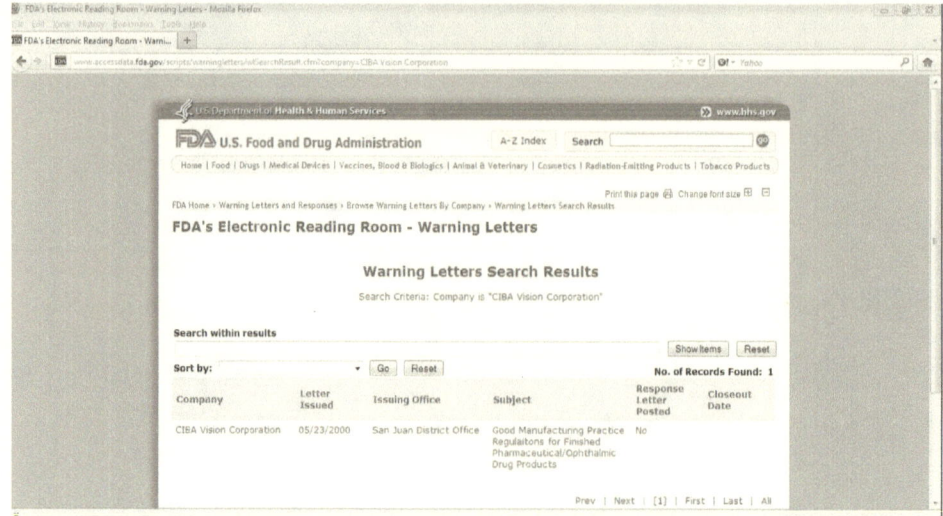

Figure 10

So, as a drug buying consumer, there are three (3) useful ways to look at Warning Letters on FDA's website. To see who is in trouble now, look at the most recent Warning Letters. For recent, but not necessarily the most recent, look at current year Warning Letters, and for older letters, search back by year. Finally, there is the option to check out a specific company.

Warning Letter listings and company listings are by no means limited to drug products. They include biological (blood) products, medical devices (catheters, stents, pacemakers, monitors, diagnostics, surgical supplies such as artificial knees and hips, and many others), foods, cosmetics, hospitals, clinical researchers and testing laboratories for example. The amount of information posted on FDAs Warning Letters section of their website is almost endless.

So what's next? What about enforcement reports? While Warning Letters are a great barometer of company practices in terms of GMP compliance and how they operate, Enforcement Reports list recalls, which to the consumer is of more immediate value. To access FDA Enforcement Reports, Referring to Figure 1, under **Approvals & Clearances**, click on Enforcement Reports. The following screen appears.

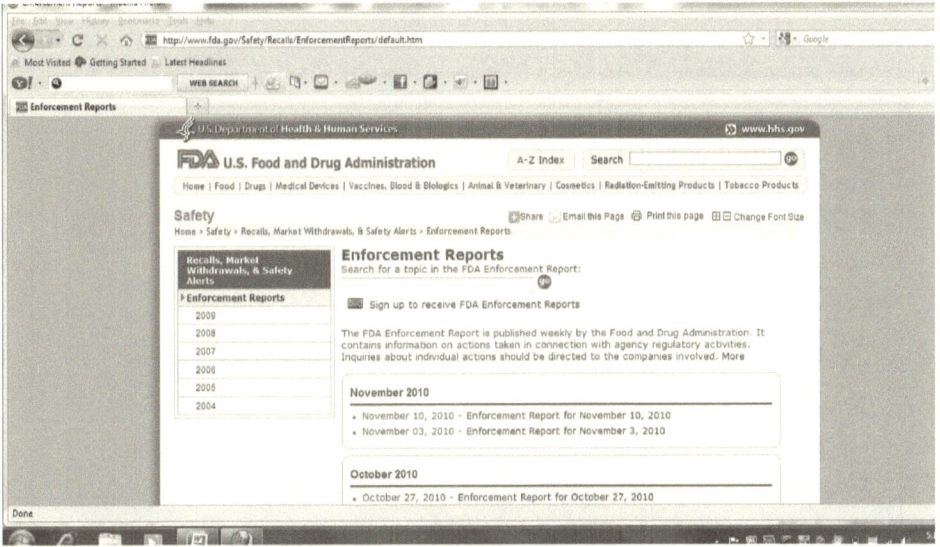

Figure 11

Looking at the lower right side of the screen under dates for the current month (the above shows November 2010 which was the current month at the time of this writing), click on **"Enforcement Report for *One of the Current Dates*"** on your screen. The entire enforcement report for that week is displayed. Categories include cosmetics, foods, drugs, medical devices, biologics and veterinary drugs. Each category is listed by class, with Class I being the most serious, then Class II and finally the least serious, Class III. Excerpts from the Enforcement Report for August 25, 2010 are shown below. As an exercise, try pulling up the Enforcement Report for August 25, 2010 by clicking on 2010 and then scrolling down to the month of august. Once the August 25 report is located, simply click on it to pull it up.

Excerpt 1

RECALLS AND FIELD CORRECTIONS: FOODS - CLASS I

PRODUCT

Romaine Lettuce in bulk bins. Recall # F-2653-2010

CODE

Lot numbers 2-6E (Y267), 2-6M (Y266), 2-6W (Y264)1

RECALLING FIRM/MANUFACTURER

Andrew Smith Co., Salinas, CA, via e-mail and telephone on May 7, 2010. FDA Initiated recall is ongoing.

REASON

Product may be contaminated with e.coli O145. Related to Freshway Foods Recall, linked to outbreak.

VOLUME OF PRODUCT IN COMMERCE

1,331 cases

DISTRIBUTION

OK, MA

PRODUCT

Ice cream in 3 lb tubs with label reading in part: "DENALI BEAR CLAW Ingredients: milkfat and nonfat milk, corn syrup, sugar, buttermilk, butter, milk, cashews. Allergen Alert: Produced in plant that uses eggs, gluten, peanuts and other nuts. Item Number: 061041. Recall # F-2666-2010

CODE

Lot code: "10124" Breakdown: "10"=year 2010, "124"=Julian date (5/4/2110) No Expiration Date

RECALLING FIRM/MANUFACTURER

Oregon Ice Cream, LLC, Eugene, OR, by letters and press release on July 23, 2010. Firm initiated recall is ongoing.

REASON

Product contains undeclared peanut allergen.

VOLUME OF PRODUCT IN COMMERCE

641 3 gallon containers

DISTRIBUTION

Nationwide

Excerpt 2

RECALLS AND FIELD CORRECTIONS: DRUGS - CLASS II

PRODUCT
LORAZEPAM Injection, USP 2 mg/mL. 10 - 1mL vials, Rx only, For IM or IV use, NDC 0409-6778-02. Recall # D-769-2010
CODE
Lot Number: 88643EV01
RECALLING FIRM/MANUFACTURER
Recalling Firm: AmeriSource Bergen, Chesterbrook, PA, by letter and follow up telephone on July 7, 2010.
Manufacturer: Hospira Inc., Lake Forest, IL. Firm initiated recall is ongoing.
REASON
Temperature Deviation; product had not been stored according to manufacturer's labeled temperature requirements prior to distribution.
VOLUME OF PRODUCT IN COMMERCE
163 units
DISTRIBUTION
FL

PRODUCT
Kit for the Preparation of Technetium Tc99m Pentetate Injection (DTPA), 10 mL vial, a) 5 vial kits (NDC 45567-0010-1), b) 30 vial kits (NDC 45567-0010-2), Rx only. Recall # D-770-2010
CODE
Lot #s: 2414, Exp. Sept 30, 2010; 2416 Exp. June 30, 2011
RECALLING FIRM/MANUFACTURER
Pharmalucence, Inc., Bedford, MA, by email and letters on August 5, 2010. Firm initiated recall is ongoing.
REASON
Product Lacks Stability: Technetium Tc99m Pentetate Injection does not maintain 90% Radiochemical Purity (RCP) for up to six hours after reconstitution with up to 160 mCi of Technetium Tc99m.
VOLUME OF PRODUCT IN COMMERCE
15,595 vials
DISTRIBUTION
Nationwide, Costa Rica, Bermuda, Israel, Republic of Panama

PRODUCT
ALTACE (ramipril) capsules, 2.5 mg, 100-count bottle, Rx only; NDC 61570-111-01. Recall # D-771-2010
CODE
Lot Number 57425, Exp 10/12
RECALLING FIRM/MANUFACTURER
King Pharmaceuticals Inc., Bristol, TN, by letter dated August 2, 2010. Firm initiated recall is ongoing.
REASON
Subpotent (Single Ingredient Drug): This product is being recalled because stability samples found that it was subpotent at the 6-month time point.

Excerpt 3

RECALLS AND FIELD CORRECTIONS: BIOLOGICS - CLASS II

PRODUCT
Source Plasma. Recall # B-2042-10
CODE
Units: 0140013769, 0140013912, 0140014133, 0140014389, 0140016295, 0140016392, 0140017155, 0140017615, 0140018074, 0140018220
RECALLING FIRM/MANUFACTURER
Recalling Firm: Biomat USA, Inc., Los Angeles, CA, by facsimile on July 1, 2009.
Manufacturer: Biomat USA, Inc., Fort Smith, AR. Firm initiated recall is complete.
REASON
Blood products, collected from a donor who received a piercing and tattoo within 12
months of donation, were distributed.
VOLUME OF PRODUCT IN COMMERCE
10 units
DISTRIBUTION
Spain

PRODUCT
Source Plasma. Recall # B-2045-10
CODE

Units: 06SWIG1280, 06SWIG0699, 06SWIF8355, 06SWIF7642, 06SWIG2241, 06SWIF9846, 06SWIF9006

RECALLING FIRM/MANUFACTURER

Recalling Firm: BioLife Plasma Services LP, Deerfield, IL, by facsimile on March 5, 2007.

Manufacturer: BioLife Plasma Services LLC, Sheboygan, WI. Firm initiated recall is complete.

REASON

Blood products, collected from a donor who was incarcerated, were distributed.

VOLUME OF PRODUCT IN COMMERCE

7 units

DISTRIBUTION

Austria

PRODUCT

Platelets Pheresis Leukocytes Reduced. Recall # B-2046-10

CODE

Units: 302683420 (2 units)

RECALLING FIRM/MANUFACTURER

Recalling Firm: Blood Systems Inc., Scottsdale, AZ, by telephone on February 28, 2008.

Manufacturer: Blood Systems, Inc., Fargo, ND. Firm initiated recall is complete.

REASON

Blood products, which were labeled as leukoreduced, but were not tested to verify white blood cell count, were distributed.

Excerpt 4

RECALLS AND FIELD CORRECTIONS: DEVICES - CLASS II

PRODUCT

19" Barco MFCD 1219 (Touch Screen) + Low Profile Stand and Rack with LCD Arm Agfa's Computed Radiography Systems with NX2.X software are indicated for use in providing diagnostic quality images to aid the physician with diagnosis. Recall # Z-2100-2010

CODE

Lot: *LU8QJ000*

RECALLING FIRM/MANUFACTURER

Recalling Firm: AGFA Corp., Greenville, SC, by letter dated June 30, 2010.

Manufacturer: Agfa Healthcare Corp., Carlstadt, NJ. Firm initiated recall is ongoing.

REASON

Monitor fell from the mounting bracket used to support the monitor

VOLUME OF PRODUCT IN COMMERCE

805 units

DISTRIBUTION

Nationwide and Canada

PRODUCT

1) Merit Laureate Hydrophylic Guide Wire, Angled, Made In Ireland, CAT No: LWSTDA35180, 180cm, Sterile EO. Intended to facilitate the placement of devices during diagnostic and interventional procedures. Recall # Z-2101-2010;

2) Merit Laureate Hydrophylic Guide Wire, Angled Stiff Shaft, Made In Ireland, CAT No: LWSTFA35180, 180cm, Sterile EO. Intended to facilitate the placement of devices during diagnostic and interventional procedures. Recall # Z-2102-2010;

3) Merit Laureate Hydrophylic Guide Wire, Straight, Made In Ireland, CAT No: LWSTFS35180, 180cm, Sterile EO. Intended to facilitate the placement of devices during diagnostic and interventional procedures. Recall # Z-2103-2010;

4) Merit Laureate Hydrophylic Guide Wire, Angled, Made In Ireland, CAT No: LWSTDA35260EX, 260cm, Sterile EO. Intended to facilitate the placement of devices during diagnostic and interventional procedures. Recall # Z-2104-2010;

5) Merit Laureate Hydrophylic Guide Wire, Angled Stiff Shaft, Made In Ireland, CAT No: LWSTFA35260EX, 260cm, Sterile EO. Intended to facilitate the placement of devices during diagnostic and interventional procedures. Recall # Z-2105-2010

6) Merit Laureate Hydrophylic Guide Wire, Straight Stiff Shaft, Made in Ireland, CAT No: LWSTFS35260EX, 260cm, Sterile EO. Intended to facilitate the placement of devices during diagnostic and interventional procedures. Recall # Z-2106-2010

CODE
1) Lot Number K131823;
2) Lot Number K131824;
3) Lot Number K131832;
4) Lot Number K130761 (3 year expiry), P116003 (1 year expiry);
5) Lot Number K131835;
6) Lot Number K131837

RECALLING FIRM/MANUFACTURER
Recalling Firm: Merit Medical Systems, Inc., South Jordan, UT, by e-mail on June 28, 2010.
Manufacturer: Merit Medical Ireland Ltd., Galway, Ireland. Firm initiated recall is complete.

REASON
Guidewires have decreased lubricity at the proximal end, inhibiting proper operation.

VOLUME OF PRODUCT IN COMMERCE
964 units

DISTRIBUTION
Nationwide

The above August 25, 2010 Enforcement Report excerpts include one excerpt each for foods, drug, biologics and devices. This Enforcement Report does not include any cosmetics or seizures, but they also will appear from time to time. Weekly enforcement reports are generally published on Wednesdays.

We always hear about recalls of automobiles, children's toys, kitchen appliances and such, but you hardly ever hear about FDA-regulated industry recalls unless they are major recalls such as the salmonella problem with eggs in the summer of 2010, or the effect of the Gulf oil spill, or drugs that have serious post-market problems that must be pulled off the market. If one browses through weekly FDA Enforcement Reports, it is evident that recalls of foods, drugs, biological and devices are quite prevalent.

For drugs, as previously mentioned, recalls can be a result issues such as stability failures, labeling, mix ups, contamination and sub or super potent active ingredients.

Looking at excerpts shown for the August 25, 2020 report, note that the format for all categories and classes is the same. For each Field Correction and Recall, the following are listed:

- *PRODUCT*—product name and description.
- *CODE*—product lot number(s)
- *RECALLING FIRM/MANUFACTURER*—name of the recalling firm and manufacturer. Sometimes they are the same, sometimes not. With drugs for example, if a company that sells a drug that has its label on it, has it made by a third-party contractor, then the company whose label is on the product is responsible for the recall, not the manufacturer.
- *REASON*—the reason for the recall such as labeling errors, mix ups or contamination.
- *VOLUME OF PRODUCT IN COMMERCE*—how much product is out there that needs to be recalled?
- *DISTRIBUTION*—*where was the product distributed? Nationwide, certain states only, etc.*

Final Thoughts:

Chapter 1, "*The Basic*" presented a general look at how the pharmaceutical industry works and how it is inspected by FDA. Chapter 2, "*Truth or Consequences*" went inside the pharmaceutical industry with a look at the cost and consequences of non-compliant operating practices. Chapter 3, "*Drug Approvals and the Generic World*", described how new drugs are approved in the United States, with an emphasis on the generic drug world, focusing on the risks and shortcomings associated with generic drugs, especially with generic over the counter (OTC) drugs. Chapter 4, "*Real Generic Stories—Nilsen's Believe it or Not*" recounted six actual, real-life generic stories in order to reinforce an appreciation of what could be happening at some companies. Chapter 5, "*Active Pharmaceutical Ingredients*", presented a general look into the manufacture of active ingredients used in drug products, where they come from and how they are regulated. This chapter, Chapter 6, "Self Defense", is by far the most important chapter in terms of consumer protection.

Whereas the first five (5) chapters gave a bird's eye view inside the drug industry, Chapter 6 gives consumers the best tool available for smart drug shopping, namely FDA's weekly Warning Letter and Enforcement Reports. Check these reports each week to see which companies are being hammered by FDA for one reason or another, and to see what products have been recalled.

Oh!, by the way, the center of the FDA's home page contains the latest news and information about current events related to consumer safety. Browse those topics as well.

Although this book is primarily geared towards the drug industry, the generic industry in particular, it is worth mentioning that the weekly FDA Enforcement Report is also great for foods, biologics and medical devices as well. Each week, see if you have any of the recalled drugs in your medicine cabinet or any of the recalled foods in your kitchen cabinets or refrigerator. It's a great way to check your personal drug and food inventory against the weekly recalls. And, for biologics, see which blood supplies are no good for one reason or another.

So now, hopefully, you have an appreciation for how the U.S. drug industry works, in particular the generic world, plus consumer risks and reliability of drug products and active ingredients. This coupled with the information available on FDA's website will make you a better informed and smarter consumer of both prescription and OTC drugs.

One last thing—If you're lazy like me, and don't want to look up Warning Letters and Recalls, FDA will automatically email you these reports each week. All you have to do is click on the link provided in the email and the report pops up on your computer. I personally have been doing this for years. Here's how to set it up.

Click on www.fda.gov. Let's do Warning Letters first.

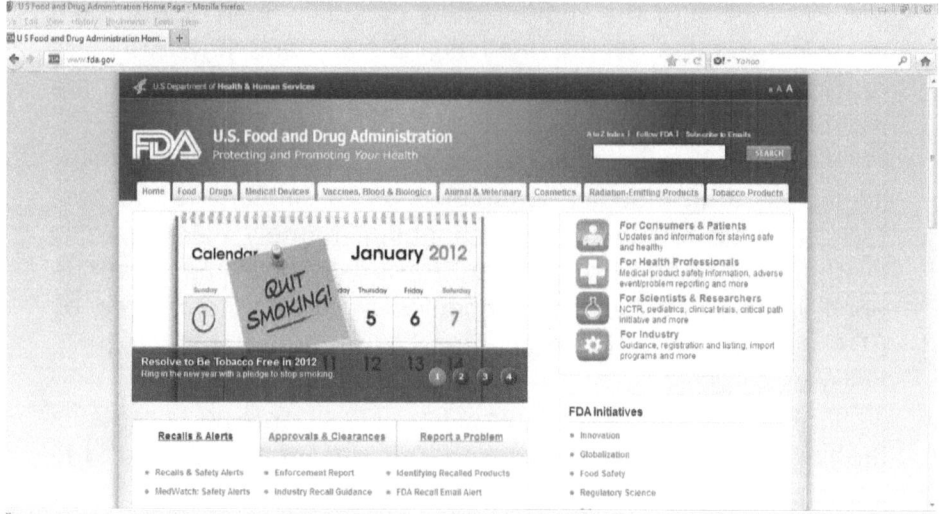

Figure 12

Bring up the FDA home page (See Figure 12)

Scroll down the home page until you get to the bottom as shown in Figure 2.

Under **Regulatory Information**, click on **"Warning Letters"**and a new screen appears (Figure 13).

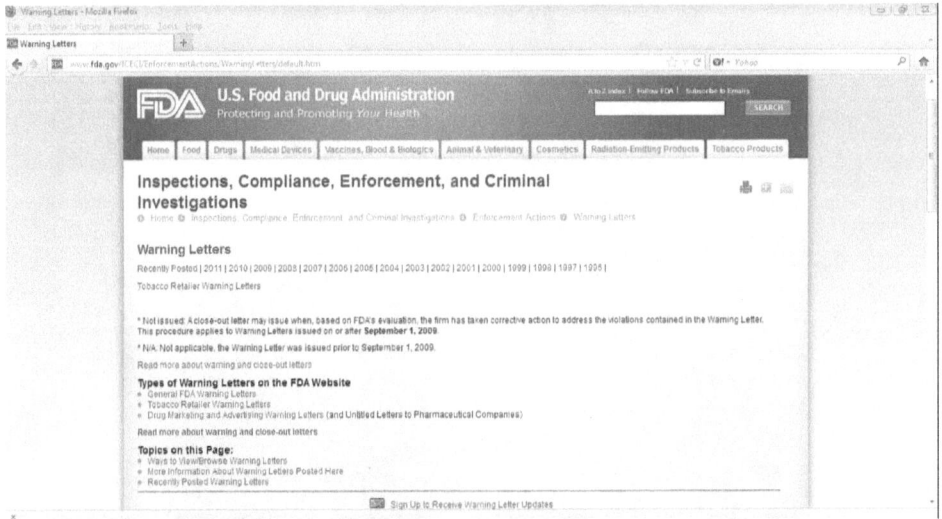

Figure 13

At the lower center part of the page, click on "**Sign Up to Receive Warning Letter Updates**" The next screen asks for your email address.

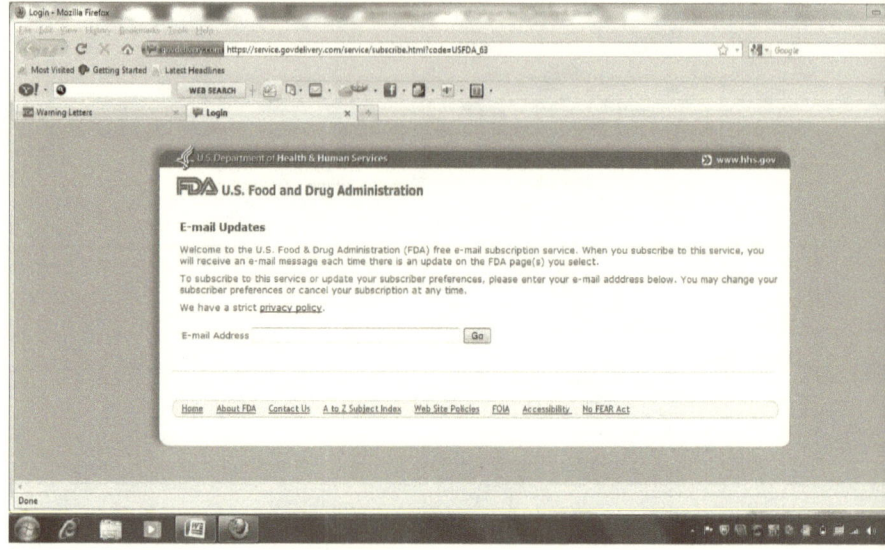

Figure 14

Just type in your email address and click **GO.** You will now get your weekly Warning Letter Reports by email.

Referring to Figure 12 (Home Page), under **Approvals & Clearances**, click on Enforcement Reports, then refer to Figure 15.

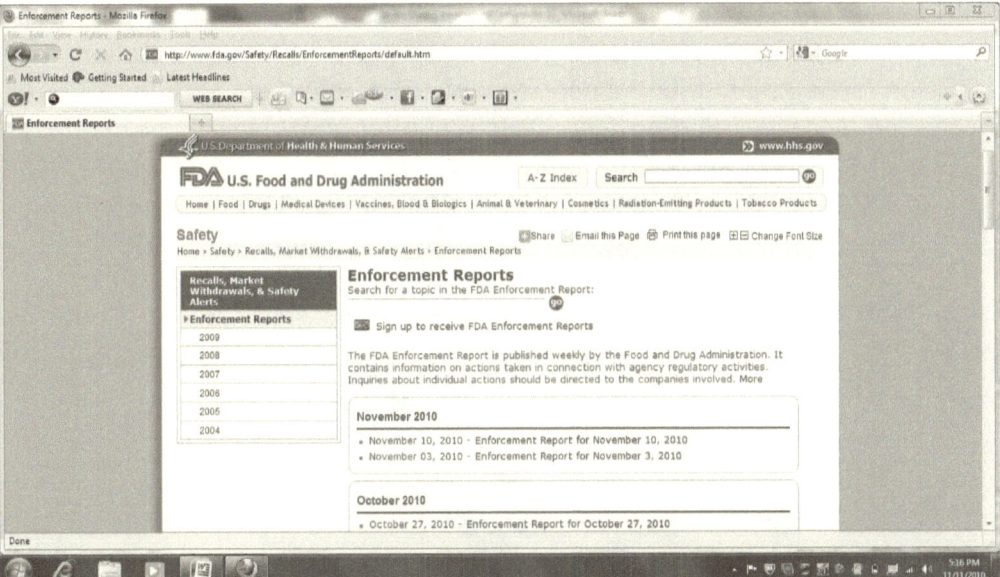

Figure 15

Click on **Sign up to receive FDA Enforcement Reports**.

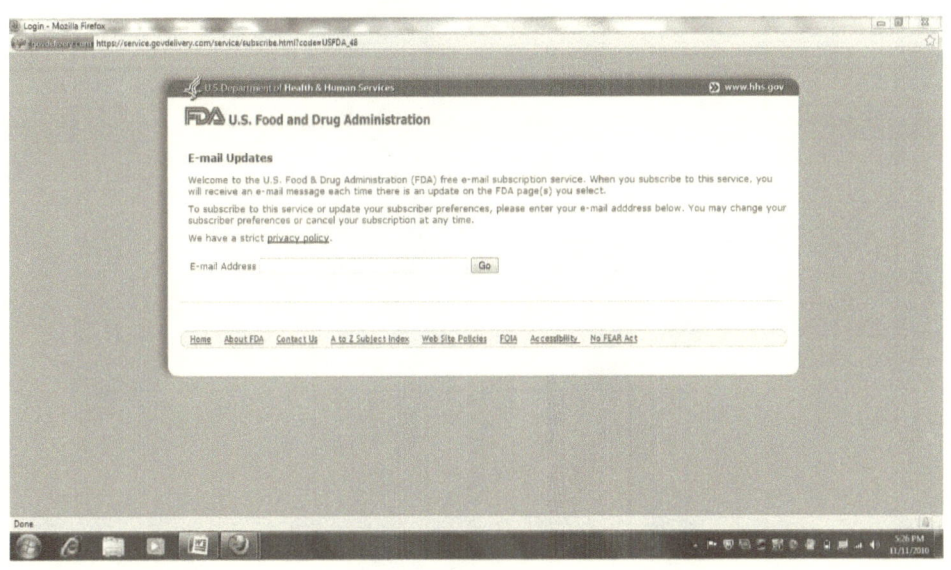

Figure 16

Now type in your email address and click **GO.** You will start getting your weekly Enforcement Reports by email.

There you have it, everything you need to navigate the world of prescription and OTC drugs, plus as a bonus, some information on foods and nutritional supplements. But before we end, here's one more for the road. The Warning Letter shown in Appendix II just another example of generic company follies. The company cited is a very large Indian-based pharmaceutical firm that has had their share of problems with FDA over the past few years. How would you feel about buying drugs that they manufacture?— no way! Well, let's take one last look. See Appendix II.

Happy hunting

Notices:

➤ Text of material from the United States Code of Federal Regulations, Title 21, is un-copyrighted material copied from the website of the U.S. Food & Drug Administration.

➤ Text of FDA Warning Letter and Enforcement Reports, in part or in their entirety, is un-copyrighted material copied from the website of the U.S. Food & Drug Administration.

➤ FDA website screen shots in Chapter 6 are un-copyrighted material copied directly from the website of the U.S. Food & Drug Administration.

➤ Cartoon at beginning of Chapter 6 licensed from www.cartoonstock.com

➤ Figure 1 in Chapter 3 courtesy of Agilent Technologies.

APPENDIX I
—
GMP REGULATIONS

TITLE 21--FOOD AND DRUGS
CHAPTER I--FOOD AND DRUG ADMINISTRATION
DEPARTMENT OF HEALTH AND HUMAN SERVICES
SUBCHAPTER C--DRUGS: GENERAL

PART 211   CURRENT GOOD MANUFACTURING PRACTICE
FOR FINISHED PHARMACEUTICALS

Subpart A--General Provisions

Sec. 211.1 Scope.

(a) The regulations in this part contain the minimum current good manufacturing practice for preparation of drug products for administration to humans or animals.

(b) The current good manufacturing practice regulations in this chapter as they pertain to drug products; in parts 600 through 680 of this chapter, as they pertain to drugs that are also biological products for human use; and in part 1271 of this chapter, as they are applicable to drugs that are also human cells, tissues, and cellular and tissue-based products (HCT/Ps) and that are drugs (subject to review under an application submitted under section 505 of the act or under a biological product license application under section 351 of the Public Health Service Act); supplement and do not supersede the regulations in this part unless the regulations explicitly provide otherwise. In the event of a conflict between applicable regulations in this part and in other parts of this chapter, or in parts 600 through 680 of this chapter, or in part 1271 of this chapter, the regulation specifically applicable to the drug product in question shall supersede the more general.

(c) Pending consideration of a proposed exemption, published in theFederal Registerof September 29, 1978, the requirements in this part shall not be enforced for OTC drug products if the products and all their ingredients are ordinarily marketed and consumed as human foods, and which products may also fall within the legal definition of drugs by virtue of their intended use. Therefore, until further notice, regulations under part 110 of this chapter, and where applicable, parts 113 to 129 of this chapter, shall be applied in determining whether these OTC drug products that are also foods are manufactured, processed, packed, or held under current good manufacturing practice.

Link to an amendment published at 74 FR 65431, Dec. 10, 2009.

[43 FR 45077, Sept. 29, 1978, as amended at 62 FR 66522, Dec. 19, 1997; 69 FR 29828, May 25, 2004]

Sec. 211.3 Definitions.

The definitions set forth in 210.3 of this chapter apply in this part.

Subpart B--Organization and Personnel

Sec. 211.22 Responsibilities of quality control unit.

(a) There shall be a quality control unit that shall have the responsibility and authority to approve or reject all components, drug product containers, closures, in-process materials, packaging material, labeling, and drug products, and the authority to review production records to assure that no errors have occurred or, if errors have occurred, that they have been fully investigated. The quality control unit shall be responsible for approving or rejecting drug products manufactured, processed, packed, or held under contract by another company.

(b) Adequate laboratory facilities for the testing and approval (or rejection) of components, drug product containers, closures, packaging materials, in-process materials, and drug products shall be available to the quality control unit.

(c) The quality control unit shall have the responsibility for approving or rejecting all procedures or specifications impacting on the identity, strength, quality, and purity of the drug product.

(d) The responsibilities and procedures applicable to the quality control unit shall be in writing; such written procedures shall be followed.

Sec. 211.25 Personnel qualifications.

(a) Each person engaged in the manufacture, processing, packing, or holding of a drug product shall have education, training, and experience, or any combination thereof, to enable that person to perform the assigned functions. Training shall be in the particular operations that the employee performs and in current good manufacturing practice (including the current good manufacturing practice regulations in this chapter and written procedures required by these regulations) as they relate to the employee's functions. Training in current good manufacturing practice shall be conducted by qualified individuals on a continuing basis and with sufficient frequency to assure that employees remain familiar with CGMP requirements applicable to them.

(b) Each person responsible for supervising the manufacture, processing, packing, or holding of a drug product shall have the education, training, and experience, or any combination thereof, to perform assigned functions in such a manner as to provide assurance that the drug product has the safety, identity, strength, quality, and purity that it purports or is represented to possess.

(c) There shall be an adequate number of qualified personnel to perform and supervise the manufacture, processing, packing, or holding of each drug product.

Sec. 211.28 Personnel responsibilities.

(a) Personnel engaged in the manufacture, processing, packing, or holding of a drug product shall wear clean clothing appropriate for the duties they perform. Protective apparel, such as head, face, hand, and arm coverings, shall be worn as necessary to protect drug products from contamination.

(b) Personnel shall practice good sanitation and health habits.

(c) Only personnel authorized by supervisory personnel shall enter those areas of the buildings and facilities designated as limited-access areas.

(d) Any person shown at any time (either by medical examination or supervisory observation) to have an apparent illness or open lesions that may adversely affect the safety or quality of drug products shall be excluded from direct contact with components, drug product containers, closures, in-process materials, and drug products until the condition is corrected or determined by competent medical personnel not to jeopardize the safety or quality of drug products. All personnel shall be instructed to report to supervisory personnel any health conditions that may have an adverse effect on drug products.

Sec. 211.34 Consultants.

Consultants advising on the manufacture, processing, packing, or holding of drug products shall have sufficient education, training, and experience, or any combination thereof, to advise on the subject for which they are retained. Records shall be maintained stating the name, address, and qualifications of any consultants and the type of service they provide.

Subpart C--Buildings and Facilities

Sec. 211.42 Design and construction features.

(a) Any building or buildings used in the manufacture, processing, packing, or holding of a drug product shall be of suitable size, construction and location to facilitate cleaning, maintenance, and proper operations.

(b) Any such building shall have adequate space for the orderly placement of equipment and materials to prevent mixups between different components, drug product containers, closures, labeling, in-process materials, or drug products, and to prevent contamination. The flow of components, drug product containers, closures, labeling, in-process materials, and drug products through the building or buildings shall be designed to prevent contamination.

(c) Operations shall be performed within specifically defined areas of adequate size. There shall be separate or defined areas or such other control systems for the firm's operations as are necessary to prevent contamination or mixups during the course of the following procedures:

(1) Receipt, identification, storage, and withholding from use of components, drug product containers, closures, and labeling, pending the appropriate sampling, testing, or examination by the quality control unit before release for manufacturing or packaging;

(2) Holding rejected components, drug product containers, closures, and labeling before disposition;

(3) Storage of released components, drug product containers, closures, and labeling;

(4) Storage of in-process materials;

(5) Manufacturing and processing operations;

(6) Packaging and labeling operations;

(7) Quarantine storage before release of drug products;

(8) Storage of drug products after release;

(9) Control and laboratory operations;

(10) Aseptic processing, which includes as appropriate:

(i) Floors, walls, and ceilings of smooth, hard surfaces that are easily cleanable;

(ii) Temperature and humidity controls;

(iii) An air supply filtered through high-efficiency particulate air filters under positive pressure, regardless of whether flow is laminar or nonlaminar;

(iv) A system for monitoring environmental conditions;

(v) A system for cleaning and disinfecting the room and equipment to produce aseptic conditions;

(vi) A system for maintaining any equipment used to control the aseptic conditions.

(d) Operations relating to the manufacture, processing, and packing of penicillin shall be performed in facilities separate from those used for other drug products for human use.

[43 FR 45077, Sept. 29, 1978, as amended at 60 FR 4091, Jan. 20, 1995]

Sec. 211.44 Lighting.

Adequate lighting shall be provided in all areas.

Sec. 211.46 Ventilation, air filtration, air heating and cooling.

(a) Adequate ventilation shall be provided.

(b) Equipment for adequate control over air pressure, micro-organisms, dust, humidity, and temperature shall be provided when appropriate for the manufacture, processing, packing, or holding of a drug product.

(c) Air filtration systems, including prefilters and particulate matter air filters, shall be used when appropriate on air supplies to production areas. If air is recirculated to production areas, measures shall be taken to control recirculation of dust from production. In areas where air contamination occurs during production, there shall be adequate exhaust systems or other systems adequate to control contaminants.

(d) Air-handling systems for the manufacture, processing, and packing of penicillin shall be completely separate from those for other drug products for human use.

Sec. 211.48 Plumbing.

(a) Potable water shall be supplied under continuous positive pressure in a plumbing system free of defects that could contribute contamination to any drug product. Potable water shall meet the standards prescribed in the Environmental Protection Agency's Primary Drinking Water Regulations set forth in 40 CFR part 141. Water not meeting such standards shall not be permitted in the potable water system.

(b) Drains shall be of adequate size and, where connected directly to a sewer, shall be provided with an air break or other mechanical device to prevent back-siphonage.

[43 FR 45077, Sept. 29, 1978, as amended at 48 FR 11426, Mar. 18, 1983]

Sec. 211.50 Sewage and refuse.

Sewage, trash, and other refuse in and from the building and immediate premises shall be disposed of in a safe and sanitary manner.

Sec. 211.52 Washing and toilet facilities.

Adequate washing facilities shall be provided, including hot and cold water, soap or detergent, air driers or single-service towels, and clean toilet facilities easily accesible to working areas.

Sec. 211.56 Sanitation.

(a) Any building used in the manufacture, processing, packing, or holding of a drug product shall be maintained in a clean and sanitary condition, Any such building shall be free of infestation by rodents, birds, insects, and other vermin (other than laboratory animals). Trash and organic waste matter shall be held and disposed of in a timely and sanitary manner.

(b) There shall be written procedures assigning responsibility for sanitation and describing in sufficient detail the cleaning schedules, methods, equipment, and materials to be used in cleaning the buildings and facilities; such written procedures shall be followed.

(c) There shall be written procedures for use of suitable rodenticides, insecticides, fungicides, fumigating agents, and cleaning and sanitizing agents. Such written procedures shall be designed to prevent the contamination of equipment, components, drug product containers, closures, packaging, labeling materials, or drug products and shall be followed. Rodenticides, insecticides, and fungicides shall not be used unless registered and used in accordance with the Federal Insecticide, Fungicide, and Rodenticide Act (7 U.S.C. 135).

(d) Sanitation procedures shall apply to work performed by contractors or temporary employees as well as work performed by full-time employees during the ordinary course of operations.

Sec. 211.58 Maintenance.

Any building used in the manufacture, processing, packing, or holding of a drug product shall be maintained in a good state of repair.

Subpart D--Equipment

Sec. 211.63 Equipment design, size, and location.

Equipment used in the manufacture, processing, packing, or holding of a drug product shall be of appropriate design, adequate size, and suitably located to facilitate operations for its intended use and for its cleaning and maintenance.

Sec. 211.65 Equipment construction.

(a) Equipment shall be constructed so that surfaces that contact components, in-process materials, or drug products shall not be reactive, additive, or absorptive so as to alter the safety, identity, strength, quality, or purity of the drug product beyond the official or other established requirements.

(b) Any substances required for operation, such as lubricants or coolants, shall not come into contact with components, drug product containers, closures, in-process materials, or drug products so as to alter the safety, identity, strength, quality, or purity of the drug product beyond the official or other established requirements.

Sec. 211.67 Equipment cleaning and maintenance.

(a) Equipment and utensils shall be cleaned, maintained, and, as appropriate for the nature of the drug, sanitized and/or sterilized at appropriate intervals to prevent malfunctions or contamination that would alter the safety, identity, strength, quality, or purity of the drug product beyond the official or other established requirements.

(b) Written procedures shall be established and followed for cleaning and maintenance of equipment, including utensils, used in the manufacture, processing, packing, or holding of a drug product. These procedures shall include, but are not necessarily limited to, the following:

(1) Assignment of responsibility for cleaning and maintaining equipment;

(2) Maintenance and cleaning schedules, including, where appropriate, sanitizing schedules;

(3) A description in sufficient detail of the methods, equipment, and materials used in cleaning and maintenance operations, and the methods of disassembling and reassembling equipment as necessary to assure proper cleaning and maintenance;

(4) Removal or obliteration of previous batch identification;

(5) Protection of clean equipment from contamination prior to use;

(6) Inspection of equipment for cleanliness immediately before use.

(c) Records shall be kept of maintenance, cleaning, sanitizing, and inspection as specified in 211.180 and 211.182.

[43 FR 45077, Sept. 29, 1978, as amended at 73 FR 51931, Sept. 8, 2008]

Sec. 211.68 Automatic, mechanical, and electronic equipment.

(a) Automatic, mechanical, or electronic equipment or other types of equipment, including computers, or related systems that will perform a function satisfactorily, may be used in the manufacture, processing, packing, and holding of a drug product. If such equipment is so used, it shall be routinely calibrated, inspected, or checked according to a written program designed to assure proper performance. Written records of those calibration checks and inspections shall be maintained.

(b) Appropriate controls shall be exercised over computer or related systems to assure that changes in master production and control records or other records are instituted only by authorized personnel. Input to and output from the computer or related system of formulas or other records or data shall be checked for accuracy. The degree and frequency of input/output verification shall be based on the complexity and reliability of the computer or related system. A backup file of data entered into the computer or related system shall be maintained except where certain data, such as calculations performed in connection with laboratory analysis, are eliminated by computerization or other automated processes. In such instances a written record of the program shall be maintained along with appropriate validation data. Hard copy or alternative systems, such as duplicates, tapes, or microfilm, designed to assure that backup data are exact and complete and that it is secure from alteration, inadvertent erasures, or loss shall be maintained.

(c) Such automated equipment used for performance of operations addressed by 211.101(c) or (d), 211.103, 211.182, or 211.188(b)(11) can satisfy the requirements included in those sections relating to the performance of an operation by one person and checking by another person if such equipment is used in conformity with this section, and one person checks that the equipment properly performed the operation.

[43 FR 45077, Sept. 29, 1978, as amended at 60 FR 4091, Jan. 20, 1995; 73 FR 51932, Sept. 8, 2008]

Sec. 211.72 Filters.

Filters for liquid filtration used in the manufacture, processing, or packing of injectable drug products intended for human use shall not release fibers into such products. Fiber-releasing filters may be used when it is not possible to manufacture such products without the use of these filters. If use of a fiber-releasing filter is necessary, an additional nonfiber-releasing filter having a maximum nominal pore size rating of 0.2 micron (0.45 micron if the manufacturing conditions so dictate) shall subsequently be used to reduce the content of particles in the injectable drug product. The use of an asbestos-containing filter is prohibited.

[73 FR 51932, Sept. 8, 2008]

Subpart E--Control of Components and Drug Product Containers and Closures

Sec. 211.80 General requirements.

(a) There shall be written procedures describing in sufficient detail the receipt, identification, storage, handling, sampling, testing, and approval or rejection of components and drug product containers and closures; such written procedures shall be followed.

(b) Components and drug product containers and closures shall at all times be handled and stored in a manner to prevent contamination.

(c) Bagged or boxed components of drug product containers, or closures shall be stored off the floor and suitably spaced to permit cleaning and inspection.

(d) Each container or grouping of containers for components or drug product containers, or closures shall be identified with a distinctive code for each lot in each shipment received. This code shall be used in recording the disposition of each lot. Each lot shall be appropriately identified as to its status (i.e., quarantined, approved, or rejected).

Sec. 211.82 Receipt and storage of untested components, drug product containers, and closures.

(a) Upon receipt and before acceptance, each container or grouping of containers of components, drug product containers, and closures shall be examined visually for appropriate labeling as to contents, container damage or broken seals, and contamination.

(b) Components, drug product containers, and closures shall be stored under quarantine until they have been tested or examined, whichever is appropriate, and released. Storage within the area shall conform to the requirements of 211.80.

Clifford L. Nilsen

[43 FR 45077, Sept. 29, 1978, as amended at 73 FR 51932, Sept. 8, 2008]

Sec. 211.84 Testing and approval or rejection of components, drug product containers, and closures.

(a) Each lot of components, drug product containers, and closures shall be withheld from use until the lot has been sampled, tested, or examined, as appropriate, and released for use by the quality control unit.

(b) Representative samples of each shipment of each lot shall be collected for testing or examination. The number of containers to be sampled, and the amount of material to be taken from each container, shall be based upon appropriate criteria such as statistical criteria for component variability, confidence levels, and degree of precision desired, the past quality history of the supplier, and the quantity needed for analysis and reserve where required by 211.170.

(c) Samples shall be collected in accordance with the following procedures:

(1) The containers of components selected shall be cleaned when necessary in a manner to prevent introduction of contaminants into the component.

(2) The containers shall be opened, sampled, and resealed in a manner designed to prevent contamination of their contents and contamination of other components, drug product containers, or closures.

(3) Sterile equipment and aseptic sampling techniques shall be used when necessary.

(4) If it is necessary to sample a component from the top, middle, and bottom of its container, such sample subdivisions shall not be composited for testing.

(5) Sample containers shall be identified so that the following information can be determined: name of the material sampled, the lot number, the container from which the sample was taken, the date on which the sample was taken, and the name of the person who collected the sample.

(6) Containers from which samples have been taken shall be marked to show that samples have been removed from them.

(d) Samples shall be examined and tested as follows:

(1) At least one test shall be conducted to verify the identity of each component of a drug product. Specific identity tests, if they exist, shall be used.

(2) Each component shall be tested for conformity with all appropriate written specifications for purity, strength, and quality. In lieu of such testing by the manufacturer, a report of analysis may be accepted from the supplier of a component, provided that at least one specific identity test is conducted on such component by the manufacturer, and provided that the manufacturer establishes the reliability of the supplier's analyses through appropriate validation of the supplier's test results at appropriate intervals.

(3) Containers and closures shall be tested for conformity with all appropriate written specifications. In lieu of such testing by the manufacturer, a certificate of testing may be accepted from the supplier, provided that at least a visual identification is conducted on such containers/closures by the manufacturer and provided that the manufacturer establishes the reliability of the supplier's test results through appropriate validation of the supplier's test results at appropriate intervals.

(4) When appropriate, components shall be microscopically examined.

(5) Each lot of a component, drug product container, or closure that is liable to contamination with filth, insect infestation, or other extraneous adulterant shall be examined against established specifications for such contamination.

(6) Each lot of a component, drug product container, or closure with potential for microbiological contamination that is objectionable in view of its intended use shall be subjected to microbiological tests before use.

(e) Any lot of components, drug product containers, or closures that meets the appropriate written specifications of identity, strength, quality, and purity and related tests under paragraph (d) of this section may be approved and released for use. Any lot of such material that does not meet such specifications shall be rejected.

[43 FR 45077, Sept. 29, 1978, as amended at 63 FR 14356, Mar. 25, 1998; 73 FR 51932, Sept. 8, 2008]

Sec. 211.86 Use of approved components, drug product containers, and closures.

Components, drug product containers, and closures approved for use shall be rotated so that the oldest approved stock is used first. Deviation from this requirement is permitted if such deviation is temporary and appropriate.

Sec. 211.87 Retesting of approved components, drug product containers, and closures.

Components, drug product containers, and closures shall be retested or reexamined, as appropriate, for identity, strength, quality, and purity and approved or rejected by the quality control unit in accordance with 211.84 as necessary, e.g., after storage for long periods or after exposure to air, heat or other conditions that might adversely affect the component, drug product container, or closure.

Sec. 211.89 Rejected components, drug product containers, and closures.

Rejected components, drug product containers, and closures shall be identified and controlled under a quarantine system designed to prevent their use in manufacturing or processing operations for which they are unsuitable.

Sec. 211.94 Drug product containers and closures.

(a) Drug product containers and closures shall not be reactive, additive, or absorptive so as to alter the safety, identity, strength, quality, or purity of the drug beyond the official or established requirements.

(b) Container closure systems shall provide adequate protection against foreseeable external factors in storage and use that can cause deterioration or contamination of the drug product.

(c) Drug product containers and closures shall be clean and, where indicated by the nature of the drug, sterilized and processed to remove pyrogenic properties to assure that they are suitable for their intended use. Such depyrogenation processes shall be validated.

(d) Standards or specifications, methods of testing, and, where indicated, methods of cleaning, sterilizing, and processing to remove pyrogenic properties shall be written and followed for drug product containers and closures.

[43 FR 45077, Sept. 29, 1978, as amended at 73 FR 51932, Sept. 8, 2008]

Subpart F--Production and Process Controls

Sec. 211.100 Written procedures; deviations.

(a) There shall be written procedures for production and process control designed to assure that the drug products have the identity, strength, quality, and purity they purport or are represented to possess. Such procedures shall include all requirements in this subpart. These written procedures, including any changes, shall be drafted, reviewed, and approved by the appropriate organizational units and reviewed and approved by the quality control unit.

(b) Written production and process control procedures shall be followed in the execution of the various production and process control functions and shall be documented at the time of performance. Any deviation from the written procedures shall be recorded and justified.

Sec. 211.101 Charge-in of components.

Written production and control procedures shall include the following, which are designed to assure that the drug products produced have the identity, strength, quality, and purity they purport or are represented to possess:

(a) The batch shall be formulated with the intent to provide not less than 100 percent of the labeled or established amount of active ingredient.

(b) Components for drug product manufacturing shall be weighed, measured, or subdivided as appropriate. If a component is removed from the original container to another, the new container shall be identified with the following information:

(1) Component name or item code;

(2) Receiving or control number;

(3) Weight or measure in new container;

(4) Batch for which component was dispensed, including its product name, strength, and lot number.

(c) Weighing, measuring, or subdividing operations for components shall be adequately supervised. Each container of component dispensed to manufacturing shall be examined by a second person to assure that:

(1) The component was released by the quality control unit;

(2) The weight or measure is correct as stated in the batch production records;

(3) The containers are properly identified. If the weighing, measuring, or subdividing operations are performed by automated equipment under 211.68, only one person is needed to assure paragraphs (c)(1), (c)(2), and (c)(3) of this section.

(d) Each component shall either be added to the batch by one person and verified by a second person or, if the components are added by automated equipment under 211.68, only verified by one person.

[43 FR 45077, Sept. 29, 1978, as amended at 73 FR 51932, Sept. 8, 2008]

Sec. 211.103 Calculation of yield.

Actual yields and percentages of theoretical yield shall be determined at the conclusion of each appropriate phase of manufacturing, processing, packaging, or holding of the drug product. Such calculations shall either be performed by one person and independently verified by a second person, or, if the yield is calculated by automated equipment under 211.68, be independently verified by one person.

[73 FR 51932, Sept. 8, 2008]

Sec. 211.105 Equipment identification.

(a) All compounding and storage containers, processing lines, and major equipment used during the production of a batch of a drug product shall be properly identified at all times to indicate their contents and, when necessary, the phase of processing of the batch.

(b) Major equipment shall be identified by a distinctive identification number or code that shall be recorded in the batch production record to show the specific equipment used in the manufacture of each batch of a drug product. In cases where only one of a particular type of equipment exists in a manufacturing facility, the name of the equipment may be used in lieu of a distinctive identification number or code.

Sec. 211.110 Sampling and testing of in-process materials and drug products.

(a) To assure batch uniformity and integrity of drug products, written procedures shall be established and followed that describe the in-process controls, and tests, or examinations to be conducted on appropriate samples of in-process materials of each batch. Such control procedures shall be established to monitor the output and to validate the performance of those manufacturing processes that may be responsible for causing variability in the characteristics of in-process material and the drug product. Such control procedures shall include, but are not limited to, the following, where appropriate:

(1) Tablet or capsule weight variation;

(2) Disintegration time;

(3) Adequacy of mixing to assure uniformity and homogeneity;

(4) Dissolution time and rate;

(5) Clarity, completeness, or pH of solutions.

(6) Bioburden testing.

(b) Valid in-process specifications for such characteristics shall be consistent with drug product final specifications and shall be derived from previous acceptable process average and process variability estimates where possible and determined by the application of suitable statistical procedures where appropriate. Examination and testing of samples shall assure that the drug product and in-process material conform to specifications.

(c) In-process materials shall be tested for identity, strength, quality, and purity as appropriate, and approved or rejected by the quality control unit, during the production process, e.g., at commencement or completion of significant phases or after storage for long periods.

(d) Rejected in-process materials shall be identified and controlled under a quarantine system designed to prevent their use in manufacturing or processing operations for which they are unsuitable.

[43 FR 45077, Sept. 29, 1978, as amended at 73 FR 51932, Sept. 8, 2008]

Sec. 211.111 Time limitations on production.

When appropriate, time limits for the completion of each phase of production shall be established to assure the quality of the drug product. Deviation from established time limits may be acceptable if such deviation does not compromise the quality of the drug product. Such deviation shall be justified and documented.

Sec. 211.113 Control of microbiological contamination.

(a) Appropriate written procedures, designed to prevent objectionable microorganisms in drug products not required to be sterile, shall be established and followed.

(b) Appropriate written procedures, designed to prevent microbiological contamination of drug products purporting to be sterile, shall be established and followed. Such procedures shall include validation of all aseptic and sterilization processes.

[43 FR 45077, Sept. 29, 1978, as amended at 73 FR 51932, Sept. 8, 2008]

Sec. 211.115 Reprocessing.

(a) Written procedures shall be established and followed prescribing a system for reprocessing batches that do not conform to standards or specifications and the steps to be taken to insure that the reprocessed batches will conform with all established standards, specifications, and characteristics.

(b) Reprocessing shall not be performed without the review and approval of the quality control unit.

Subpart G--Packaging and Labeling Control

Sec. 211.122 Materials examination and usage criteria.

(a) There shall be written procedures describing in sufficient detail the receipt, identification, storage, handling, sampling, examination, and/or testing of labeling and packaging materials; such written procedures shall be followed. Labeling and packaging materials shall be representatively sampled, and examined or tested upon receipt and before use in packaging or labeling of a drug product.

(b) Any labeling or packaging materials meeting appropriate written specifications may be approved and released for use. Any labeling or packaging materials that do not meet such specifications shall be rejected to prevent their use in operations for which they are unsuitable.

(c) Records shall be maintained for each shipment received of each different labeling and packaging material indicating receipt, examination or testing, and whether accepted or rejected.

(d) Labels and other labeling materials for each different drug product, strength, dosage form, or quantity of contents shall be stored separately with suitable identification. Access to the storage area shall be limited to authorized personnel.

(e) Obsolete and outdated labels, labeling, and other packaging materials shall be destroyed.

(f) Use of gang-printed labeling for different drug products, or different strengths or net contents of the same drug product, is prohibited unless the labeling from gang-printed sheets is adequately differentiated by size, shape, or color.

(g) If cut labeling is used, packaging and labeling operations shall include one of the following special control procedures:

(1) Dedication of labeling and packaging lines to each different strength of each different drug product;

(2) Use of appropriate electronic or electromechanical equipment to conduct a 100-percent examination for correct labeling during or after completion of finishing operations; or

(3) Use of visual inspection to conduct a 100-percent examination for correct labeling during or after completion of finishing operations for hand-applied labeling. Such examination shall be performed by one person and independently verified by a second person.

(h) Printing devices on, or associated with, manufacturing lines used to imprint labeling upon the drug product unit label or case shall be monitored to assure that all imprinting conforms to the print specified in the batch production record.

[43 FR 45077, Sept. 29, 1978, as amended at 58 FR 41353, Aug. 3, 1993]

Sec. 211.125 Labeling issuance.

(a) Strict control shall be exercised over labeling issued for use in drug product labeling operations.

(b) Labeling materials issued for a batch shall be carefully examined for identity and conformity to the labeling specified in the master or batch production records.

(c) Procedures shall be used to reconcile the quantities of labeling issued, used, and returned, and shall require evaluation of discrepancies found between the quantity of drug product finished and the quantity of labeling issued when such discrepancies are outside narrow preset limits based on historical operating data. Such discrepancies shall be investigated in accordance with 211.192. Labeling reconciliation is waived for cut or roll labeling if a 100-percent examination for correct labeling is performed in accordance with 211.122(g) (2).

(d) All excess labeling bearing lot or control numbers shall be destroyed.

(e) Returned labeling shall be maintained and stored in a manner to prevent mixups and provide proper identification.

(f) Procedures shall be written describing in sufficient detail the control procedures employed for the issuance of labeling; such written procedures shall be followed.

[43 FR 45077, Sept. 29, 1978, as amended at 58 FR 41354, Aug. 3, 1993]

Sec. 211.130 Packaging and labeling operations.

There shall be written procedures designed to assure that correct labels, labeling, and packaging materials are used for drug products; such written procedures shall be followed. These procedures shall incorporate the following features:

(a) Prevention of mixups and cross-contamination by physical or spatial separation from operations on other drug products.

(b) Identification and handling of filled drug product containers that are set aside and held in unlabeled condition for future labeling operations to preclude mislabeling of individual containers, lots, or portions of lots. Identification need not be applied to each individual container but shall be sufficient to determine name, strength, quantity of contents, and lot or control number of each container.

(c) Identification of the drug product with a lot or control number that permits determination of the history of the manufacture and control of the batch.

(d) Examination of packaging and labeling materials for suitability and correctness before packaging operations, and documentation of such examination in the batch production record.

(e) Inspection of the packaging and labeling facilities immediately before use to assure that all drug products have been removed from previous operations. Inspection shall also be made to assure that packaging and labeling materials not suitable for subsequent operations have been removed. Results of inspection shall be documented in the batch production records.

[43 FR 45077, Sept. 29, 1978, as amended at 58 FR 41354, Aug. 3, 1993]

Sec. 211.132 Tamper-evident packaging requirements for over-the-counter (OTC) human drug products.

(a) *General.* The Food and Drug Administration has the authority under the Federal Food, Drug, and Cosmetic Act (the act) to establish a uniform national requirement for tamper-evident packaging of OTC drug products that will improve the security of OTC drug packaging and help assure the safety and effectiveness of OTC drug products. An OTC drug product (except a dermatological, dentifrice, insulin, or lozenge product) for retail sale that is not packaged in a tamper-resistant package or that is not properly labeled under this section is adulterated under section 501 of the act or misbranded under section 502 of the act, or both.

(b) *Requirements for tamper-evident package.* (1) Each manufacturer and packer who packages an OTC drug product (except a dermatological, dentifrice, insulin, or lozenge product) for retail sale shall package the product in a tamper-evident package, if this product is accessible to the public while held for sale. A tamper-evident package is one having one or more indicators or barriers to entry which, if breached or missing, can reasonably be expected to provide visible evidence to consumers that tampering has occurred. To reduce the likelihood of successful tampering and to increase the likelihood that consumers will discover if a product has been tampered with, the package is required to be distinctive by design or by the use of one or more indicators or barriers to entry that employ an identifying characteristic (e.g., a pattern, name, registered trademark, logo, or picture). For purposes of this section, the term "distinctive by design" means the packaging cannot be duplicated with commonly available materials or through commonly available processes. A tamper-evident package may involve an immediate-container and closure system or secondary-container or carton system or any combination of systems intended to provide a visual indication of package integrity. The tamper-evident feature shall be designed to and shall remain intact when handled in a reasonable manner during manufacture, distribution, and retail display.

(2) In addition to the tamper-evident packaging feature described in paragraph (b)(1) of this section, any two-piece, hard gelatin capsule covered by this section must be sealed using an acceptable tamper-evident technology.

(c)*Labeling.* (1) In order to alert consumers to the specific tamper-evident feature(s) used, each retail package of an OTC drug product covered by this section (except ammonia inhalant in crushable glass ampules, containers of compressed medical oxygen, or aerosol products that depend upon the power of a liquefied or compressed gas to expel the contents from the container) is required to bear a statement that:

(i) Identifies all tamper-evident feature(s) and any capsule sealing technologies used to comply with paragraph (b) of this section;

(ii) Is prominently placed on the package; and

(iii) Is so placed that it will be unaffected if the tamper-evident feature of the package is breached or missing.

(2) If the tamper-evident feature chosen to meet the requirements in paragraph (b) of this section uses an identifying characteristic, that characteristic is required to be referred to in the labeling statement. For example, the labeling statement on a bottle with a shrink band could say "For your protection, this bottle has an imprinted seal around the neck."

(d) *Request for exemptions from packaging and labeling requirements.* A manufacturer or packer may request an exemption from the packaging and labeling requirements of this section. A request for an exemption is required to be submitted in the form of a citizen petition under 10.30 of this chapter and should be clearly identified on the envelope as a "Request for Exemption from the Tamper-Evident Packaging Rule." The petition is required to contain the following:

(1) The name of the drug product or, if the petition seeks an exemption for a drug class, the name of the drug class, and a list of products within that class.

(2) The reasons that the drug product's compliance with the tamper-evident packaging or labeling requirements of this section is unnecessary or cannot be achieved.

(3) A description of alternative steps that are available, or that the petitioner has already taken, to reduce the likelihood that the product or drug class will be the subject of malicious adulteration.

(4) Other information justifying an exemption.

(e) *OTC drug products subject to approved new drug applications.* Holders of approved new drug applications for OTC drug products are required under 314.70 of this chapter to provide the agency with notification of changes in packaging and labeling to comply with the requirements of this section. Changes in packaging and labeling required by this regulation may be made before FDA approval, as provided under 314.70(c) of this chapter. Manufacturing changes by which capsules are to be sealed require prior FDA approval under 314.70(b) of this chapter.

(f) *Poison Prevention Packaging Act of 1970.* This section does not affect any requirements for "special packaging" as defined under 310.3(l) of this chapter and required under the Poison Prevention Packaging Act of 1970.

[54 FR 5228, Feb. 2, 1989, as amended at 63 FR 59470, Nov. 4, 1998]

Sec. 211.134 Drug product inspection.

(a) Packaged and labeled products shall be examined during finishing operations to provide assurance that containers and packages in the lot have the correct label.

(b) A representative sample of units shall be collected at the completion of finishing operations and shall be visually examined for correct labeling.

(c) Results of these examinations shall be recorded in the batch production or control records.

Sec. 211.137 Expiration dating.

(a) To assure that a drug product meets applicable standards of identity, strength, quality, and purity at the time of use, it shall bear an expiration date determined by appropriate stability testing described in 211.166.

(b) Expiration dates shall be related to any storage conditions stated on the labeling, as determined by stability studies described in 211.166.

(c) If the drug product is to be reconstituted at the time of dispensing, its labeling shall bear expiration information for both the reconstituted and unreconstituted drug products.

(d) Expiration dates shall appear on labeling in accordance with the requirements of 201.17 of this chapter.

(e) Homeopathic drug products shall be exempt from the requirements of this section.

(f) Allergenic extracts that are labeled "No U.S. Standard of Potency" are exempt from the requirements of this section.

(g) New drug products for investigational use are exempt from the requirements of this section, provided that they meet appropriate standards or specifications as demonstrated by stability studies during their use in clinical investigations. Where new drug products for investigational use are to be reconstituted at the time of dispensing, their labeling shall bear expiration information for the reconstituted drug product.

(h) Pending consideration of a proposed exemption, published in theFederal Registerof September 29, 1978, the requirements in this section shall not be enforced for human OTC drug products if their labeling does not bear dosage limitations and they are stable for at least 3 years as supported by appropriate stability data.

[43 FR 45077, Sept. 29, 1978, as amended at 46 FR 56412, Nov. 17, 1981; 60 FR 4091, Jan. 20, 1995]

Subpart H--Holding and Distribution

Sec. 211.142 Warehousing procedures.

Written procedures describing the warehousing of drug products shall be established and followed. They shall include:

(a) Quarantine of drug products before release by the quality control unit.

(b) Storage of drug products under appropriate conditions of temperature, humidity, and light so that the identity, strength, quality, and purity of the drug products are not affected.

Sec. 211.150 Distribution procedures.

Written procedures shall be established, and followed, describing the distribution of drug products. They shall include:

(a) A procedure whereby the oldest approved stock of a drug product is distributed first. Deviation from this requirement is permitted if such deviation is temporary and appropriate.

(b) A system by which the distribution of each lot of drug product can be readily determined to facilitate its recall if necessary.

Subpart I--Laboratory Controls

Sec. 211.160 General requirements.

(a) The establishment of any specifications, standards, sampling plans, test procedures, or other laboratory control mechanisms required by this subpart, including any change in such specifications, standards, sampling plans, test procedures, or other laboratory control mechanisms, shall be drafted by the appropriate organizational unit and reviewed and approved by the quality control unit. The requirements in this subpart shall be followed and shall be documented at the time of performance. Any deviation from the written specifications, standards, sampling plans, test procedures, or other laboratory control mechanisms shall be recorded and justified.

(b) Laboratory controls shall include the establishment of scientifically sound and appropriate specifications, standards, sampling plans, and test procedures designed to assure that components, drug product containers, closures, in-process materials, labeling, and drug products conform to appropriate standards of identity, strength, quality, and purity. Laboratory controls shall include:

(1) Determination of conformity to applicable written specifications for the acceptance of each lot within each shipment of components, drug product containers, closures, and labeling used in the manufacture, processing, packing, or holding of drug products. The specifications shall include a description of the sampling and testing procedures used. Samples shall be representative and adequately identified. Such procedures shall also require appropriate retesting of any component, drug product container, or closure that is subject to deterioration.

(2) Determination of conformance to written specifications and a description of sampling and testing procedures

for in-process materials. Such samples shall be representative and properly identified.

(3) Determination of conformance to written descriptions of sampling procedures and appropriate specifications for drug products. Such samples shall be representative and properly identified.

(4) The calibration of instruments, apparatus, gauges, and recording devices at suitable intervals in accordance with an established written program containing specific directions, schedules, limits for accuracy and precision, and provisions for remedial action in the event accuracy and/or precision limits are not met. Instruments, apparatus, gauges, and recording devices not meeting established specifications shall not be used.

[43 FR 45077, Sept. 29, 1978, as amended at 73 FR 51932, Sept. 8, 2008]

Sec. 211.165 Testing and release for distribution.

(a) For each batch of drug product, there shall be appropriate laboratory determination of satisfactory conformance to final specifications for the drug product, including the identity and strength of each active ingredient, prior to release. Where sterility and/or pyrogen testing are conducted on specific batches of shortlived radiopharmaceuticals, such batches may be released prior to completion of sterility and/or pyrogen testing, provided such testing is completed as soon as possible.

(b) There shall be appropriate laboratory testing, as necessary, of each batch of drug product required to be free of objectionable microorganisms.

(c) Any sampling and testing plans shall be described in written procedures that shall include the method of sampling and the number of units per batch to be tested; such written procedure shall be followed.

(d) Acceptance criteria for the sampling and testing conducted by the quality control unit shall be adequate to assure that batches of drug products meet each appropriate specification and appropriate statistical quality control criteria as a condition for their approval and release. The statistical quality control criteria shall include appropriate acceptance levels and/or appropriate rejection levels.

(e) The accuracy, sensitivity, specificity, and reproducibility of test methods employed by the firm shall be established and documented. Such validation and documentation may be accomplished in accordance with 211.194(a)(2).

(f) Drug products failing to meet established standards or specifications and any other relevant quality control criteria shall be rejected. Reprocessing may be performed. Prior to acceptance and use, reprocessed material must meet appropriate standards, specifications, and any other relevant critieria.

Sec. 211.166 Stability testing.

(a) There shall be a written testing program designed to assess the stability characteristics of drug products. The results of such stability testing shall be used in determining appropriate storage conditions and expiration dates. The written program shall be followed and shall include:

(1) Sample size and test intervals based on statistical criteria for each attribute examined to assure valid estimates of stability;

(2) Storage conditions for samples retained for testing;

(3) Reliable, meaningful, and specific test methods;

(4) Testing of the drug product in the same container-closure system as that in which the drug product is marketed;

(5) Testing of drug products for reconstitution at the time of dispensing (as directed in the labeling) as well as after they are reconstituted.

(b) An adequate number of batches of each drug product shall be tested to determine an appropriate expiration date and a record of such data shall be maintained. Accelerated studies, combined with basic stability information on the components, drug products, and container-closure system, may be used to support tentative expiration dates provided full shelf life studies are not available and are being conducted. Where data from accelerated studies are used to project a tentative expiration date that is beyond a date supported by actual shelf life studies, there must be stability studies conducted, including drug product testing at appropriate intervals, until the tentative expiration date is verified or the appropriate expiration date determined.

(c) For homeopathic drug products, the requirements of this section are as follows:

(1) There shall be a written assessment of stability based at least on testing or examination of the drug product for compatibility of the ingredients, and based on marketing experience with the drug product to indicate that there is no degradation of the product for the normal or expected period of use.

(2) Evaluation of stability shall be based on the same container-closure system in which the drug product is being marketed.

(d) Allergenic extracts that are labeled "No U.S. Standard of Potency" are exempt from the requirements of this section.

[43 FR 45077, Sept. 29, 1978, as amended at 46 FR 56412, Nov. 17, 1981]

Sec. 211.167 Special testing requirements.

(a) For each batch of drug product purporting to be sterile and/or pyrogen-free, there shall be appropriate laboratory testing to determine conformance to such requirements. The test procedures shall be in writing and shall be followed.

(b) For each batch of ophthalmic ointment, there shall be appropriate testing to determine conformance to specifications regarding the presence of foreign particles and harsh or abrasive substances. The test procedures shall be in writing and shall be followed.

(c) For each batch of controlled-release dosage form, there shall be appropriate laboratory testing to determine conformance to the specifications for the rate of release of each active ingredient. The test procedures shall be in writing and shall be followed.

Sec. 211.170 Reserve samples.

(a) An appropriately identified reserve sample that is representative of each lot in each shipment of each active ingredient shall be retained. The reserve sample consists of at least twice the quantity necessary for all tests required to determine whether the active ingredient meets its established specifications, except for sterility and pyrogen testing. The retention time is as follows:

(1) For an active ingredient in a drug product other than those described in paragraphs (a) (2) and (3) of this section, the reserve sample shall be retained for 1 year after the expiration date of the last lot of the drug product containing the active ingredient.

(2) For an active ingredient in a radioactive drug product, except for nonradioactive reagent kits, the reserve sample shall be retained for:

(i) Three months after the expiration date of the last lot of the drug product containing the active ingredient if the expiration dating period of the drug product is 30 days or less; or

(ii) Six months after the expiration date of the last lot of the drug product containing the active ingredient if the expiration dating period of the drug product is more than 30 days.

(3) For an active ingredient in an OTC drug product that is exempt from bearing an expiration date under 211.137, the reserve sample shall be retained for 3 years after distribution of the last lot of the drug product containing the active ingredient.

(b) An appropriately identified reserve sample that is representative of each lot or batch of drug product shall be retained and stored under conditions consistent with product labeling. The reserve sample shall be stored in the same immediate container-closure system in which the drug product is marketed or in one that has essentially the same characteristics. The reserve sample consists of at least twice the quantity necessary to perform all the required tests, except those for sterility and pyrogens. Except for those for drug products described in paragraph (b)(2) of this section, reserve samples from representative sample lots or batches selected by acceptable statistical procedures shall be examined visually at least once a year for evidence of deterioration unless visual examination would affect the integrity of the reserve sample. Any evidence of reserve sample deterioration shall be investigated in accordance with 211.192. The results of the examination shall be recorded and maintained with other stability data on the drug product. Reserve samples of compressed medical gases need not be retained. The retention time is as follows:

(1) For a drug product other than those described in paragraphs (b) (2) and (3) of this section, the reserve sample shall be retained for 1 year after the expiration date of the drug product.

(2) For a radioactive drug product, except for nonradioactive reagent kits, the reserve sample shall be retained for:

(i) Three months after the expiration date of the drug product if the expiration dating period of the drug product is 30 days or less; or

(ii) Six months after the expiration date of the drug product if the expiration dating period of the drug product is more than 30 days.

(3) For an OTC drug product that is exempt for bearing an expiration date under 211.137, the reserve sample must be retained for 3 years after the lot or batch of drug product is distributed.

[48 FR 13025, Mar. 29, 1983, as amended at 60 FR 4091, Jan. 20, 1995]

Sec. 211.173 Laboratory animals.

Animals used in testing components, in-process materials, or drug products for compliance with established specifications shall be maintained and controlled in a manner that assures their suitability for their intended use. They shall be identified, and adequate records shall be maintained showing the history of their use.

Sec. 211.176 Penicillin contamination.

If a reasonable possibility exists that a non-penicillin drug product has been exposed to cross-contamination with penicillin, the non-penicillin drug product shall be tested for the presence of penicillin. Such drug product shall not be marketed if detectable levels are found when tested according to procedures specified in `Procedures for Detecting and Measuring Penicillin Contamination in Drugs,' which is incorporated by reference. Copies are available from the Division of Research and Testing (HFD-470), Center for Drug Evaluation and Research, Food and Drug Administration, 5100 Paint Branch Pkwy., College Park, MD 20740, or available for inspection at the National Archives and Records Administration (NARA). For information on the availability of this material at NARA, call 202-741-6030, or go to:*http://www.archives. gov/federal_register/code_of_federal_regulations/ibr_ locations.html.*

[43 FR 45077, Sept. 29, 1978, as amended at 47 FR 9396, Mar. 5, 1982; 50 FR 8996, Mar. 6, 1985; 55 FR 11577, Mar. 29, 1990; 66 FR 56035, Nov. 6, 2001; 69 FR 18803, Apr. 9, 2004]

Subpart J--Records and Reports

Sec. 211.180 General requirements.

(a) Any production, control, or distribution record that is required to be maintained in compliance with this part and is specifically associated with a batch of a drug product shall be retained for at least 1 year after the expiration date of the batch or, in the case of certain OTC drug products lacking expiration dating because they meet the criteria for exemption under 211.137, 3 years after distribution of the batch.

(b) Records shall be maintained for all components, drug product containers, closures, and labeling for at least 1 year after the expiration date or, in the case of certain OTC drug products lacking expiration dating because they meet the criteria for exemption under 211.137, 3 years after distribution of the last lot of drug product incorporating the component or using the container, closure, or labeling.

(c) All records required under this part, or copies of such records, shall be readily available for authorized inspection during the retention period at the establishment where the activities described in such records occurred. These records or copies thereof shall be subject to photocopying or other means of reproduction as part of such inspection. Records that can be immediately retrieved from another location by computer or other electronic means shall be considered as meeting the requirements of this paragraph.

(d) Records required under this part may be retained either as original records or as true copies such as photocopies, microfilm, microfiche, or other accurate reproductions of the original records. Where reduction techniques, such as microfilming, are used, suitable reader and photocopying equipment shall be readily available.

(e) Written records required by this part shall be maintained so that data therein can be used for evaluating, at least annually, the quality standards of each drug product to determine the need for changes in drug product specifications or manufacturing or control procedures. Written procedures shall be established and followed for such evaluations and shall include provisions for:

(1) A review of a representative number of batches, whether approved or rejected, and, where applicable, records associated with the batch.

(2) A review of complaints, recalls, returned or salvaged drug products, and investigations conducted under 211.192 for each drug product.

(f) Procedures shall be established to assure that the responsible officials of the firm, if they are not personally involved in or immediately aware of such actions, are notified in writing of any investigations conducted under 211.198, 211.204, or 211.208 of these regulations, any recalls, reports of inspectional observations issued by the Food and Drug Administration, or any regulatory actions relating to good manufacturing practices brought by the Food and Drug Administration.

[43 FR 45077, Sept. 29, 1978, as amended at 60 FR 4091, Jan. 20, 1995]

Sec. 211.182 Equipment cleaning and use log.

A written record of major equipment cleaning, maintenance (except routine maintenance such as lubrication and adjustments), and use shall be included in individual equipment logs that show the date, time, product, and lot number of each batch processed. If equipment is dedicated to manufacture of one product, then individual equipment logs are not required, provided that lots or batches of such product follow in numerical order and are manufactured in numerical sequence. In cases where dedicated equipment is employed, the records of cleaning, maintenance, and use shall be part of the batch record. The persons performing and double-checking the cleaning and maintenance (or, if the cleaning and maintenance is performed using automated equipment under 211.68, just the person verifying the cleaning and maintenance done by the automated equipment) shall date and sign or initial the log indicating that the work was performed. Entries in the log shall be in chronological order.

[73 FR 51933, Sept. 8, 2008]

Sec. 211.184 Component, drug product container, closure, and labeling records.

These records shall include the following:

(a) The identity and quantity of each shipment of each lot of components, drug product containers, closures, and labeling; the name of the supplier; the supplier's lot number(s) if known; the receiving code as specified in 211.80; and the date of receipt. The name and location of the prime manufacturer, if different from the supplier, shall be listed if known.

(b) The results of any test or examination performed (including those performed as required by 211.82(a), 211.84(d), or 211.122(a)) and the conclusions derived therefrom.

(c) An individual inventory record of each component, drug product container, and closure and, for each component, a reconciliation of the use of each lot of such component. The inventory record shall contain sufficient information to allow determination of any batch or lot of drug product associated with the use of each component, drug product container, and closure.

(d) Documentation of the examination and review of labels and labeling for conformity with established specifications in accord with 211.122(c) and 211.130(c).

(e) The disposition of rejected components, drug product containers, closure, and labeling.

Sec. 211.186 Master production and control records.

(a) To assure uniformity from batch to batch, master production and control records for each drug product, including each batch size thereof, shall be prepared, dated, and signed (full signature, handwritten) by one person and independently checked, dated, and signed by a second person. The preparation of master production and control records shall be described in a written procedure and such written procedure shall be followed.

(b) Master production and control records shall include:

(1) The name and strength of the product and a description of the dosage form;

(2) The name and weight or measure of each active ingredient per dosage unit or per unit of weight or measure of the drug product, and a statement of the total weight or measure of any dosage unit;

(3) A complete list of components designated by names or codes sufficiently specific to indicate any special quality characteristic;

(4) An accurate statement of the weight or measure of each component, using the same weight system (metric, avoirdupois, or apothecary) for each component. Reasonable variations may be permitted, however, in the amount of components necessary for the preparation in the dosage form, provided they are justified in the master production and control records;

(5) A statement concerning any calculated excess of component;

(6) A statement of theoretical weight or measure at appropriate phases of processing;

(7) A statement of theoretical yield, including the maximum and minimum percentages of theoretical yield beyond which investigation according to 211.192 is required;

(8) A description of the drug product containers, closures, and packaging materials, including a specimen or copy of each label and all other labeling signed and dated by the person or persons responsible for approval of such labeling;

(9) Complete manufacturing and control instructions, sampling and testing procedures, specifications, special notations, and precautions to be followed.

Sec. 211.188 Batch production and control records.

Batch production and control records shall be prepared for each batch of drug product produced and shall include complete information relating to the production and control of each batch. These records shall include:

(a) An accurate reproduction of the appropriate master production or control record, checked for accuracy, dated, and signed;

(b) Documentation that each significant step in the manufacture, processing, packing, or holding of the batch was accomplished, including:

(1) Dates;

(2) Identity of individual major equipment and lines used;

(3) Specific identification of each batch of component or in-process material used;

(4) Weights and measures of components used in the course of processing;

(5) In-process and laboratory control results;

(6) Inspection of the packaging and labeling area before and after use;

(7) A statement of the actual yield and a statement of the percentage of theoretical yield at appropriate phases of processing;

(8) Complete labeling control records, including specimens or copies of all labeling used;

(9) Description of drug product containers and closures;

(10) Any sampling performed;

(11) Identification of the persons performing and directly supervising or checking each significant step in the operation, or if a significant step in the operation is performed by automated equipment under 211.68, the identification of the person checking the significant step performed by the automated equipment.

(12) Any investigation made according to 211.192.

(13) Results of examinations made in accordance with 211.134.

[43 FR 45077, Sept. 29, 1978, as amended at 73 FR 51933, Sept. 8, 2008]

Sec. 211.192 Production record review.

All drug product production and control records, including those for packaging and labeling, shall be reviewed and approved by the quality control unit to determine compliance with all established, approved written procedures before a batch is released or distributed. Any unexplained discrepancy (including a percentage of theoretical yield exceeding the maximum or minimum percentages established in master production and control records) or the failure of a batch or any of its components to meet any of its specifications shall be thoroughly investigated, whether or not the batch has already been distributed. The investigation shall extend to other batches of the same drug product and other drug products that may have been associated with the specific failure or discrepancy. A written record of the investigation shall be made and shall include the conclusions and followup.

Sec. 211.194 Laboratory records.

(a) Laboratory records shall include complete data derived from all tests necessary to assure compliance with established specifications and standards, including examinations and assays, as follows:

(1) A description of the sample received for testing with identification of source (that is, location from where sample was obtained), quantity, lot number or other distinctive code, date sample was taken, and date sample was received for testing.

(2) A statement of each method used in the testing of the sample. The statement shall indicate the location of data that establish that the methods used in the testing of the sample meet proper standards of accuracy and reliability as applied to the product tested. (If the method employed is in the current revision of the United States Pharmacopeia, National Formulary, AOAC INTERNATIONAL, Book of Methods,[1]or in other recognized standard references, or is detailed in an approved new drug application and the referenced method is not modified, a statement indicating the method and reference will suffice). The suitability of all testing methods used shall be verified under actual conditions of use.

(3) A statement of the weight or measure of sample used for each test, where appropriate.

(4) A complete record of all data secured in the course of each test, including all graphs, charts, and spectra from laboratory instrumentation, properly identified to

show the specific component, drug product container, closure, in-process material, or drug product, and lot tested.

(5) A record of all calculations performed in connection with the test, including units of measure, conversion factors, and equivalency factors.

(6) A statement of the results of tests and how the results compare with established standards of identity, strength, quality, and purity for the component, drug product container, closure, in-process material, or drug product tested.

(7) The initials or signature of the person who performs each test and the date(s) the tests were performed.

(8) The initials or signature of a second person showing that the original records have been reviewed for accuracy, completeness, and compliance with established standards.

(b) Complete records shall be maintained of any modification of an established method employed in testing. Such records shall include the reason for the modification and data to verify that the modification produced results that are at least as accurate and reliable for the material being tested as the established method.

(c) Complete records shall be maintained of any testing and standardization of laboratory reference standards, reagents, and standard solutions.

(d) Complete records shall be maintained of the periodic calibration of laboratory instruments, apparatus, gauges, and recording devices required by 211.160(b) (4).

(e) Complete records shall be maintained of all stability testing performed in accordance with 211.166.

[1]Copies may be obtained from: AOAC INTERNATIONAL, 481 North Frederick Ave., suite 500, Gaithersburg, MD 20877.

[43 FR 45077, Sept. 29, 1978, as amended at 55 FR 11577, Mar. 29, 1990; 65 FR 18889, Apr. 10, 2000; 70 FR 40880, July 15, 2005; 70 FR 67651, Nov. 8, 2005]

Sec. 211.196 Distribution records.

Distribution records shall contain the name and strength of the product and description of the dosage form, name and address of the consignee, date and quantity shipped, and lot or control number of the drug product. For compressed medical gas products, distribution records are not required to contain lot or control numbers.

[49 FR 9865, Mar. 16, 1984]

Sec. 211.198 Complaint files.

(a) Written procedures describing the handling of all written and oral complaints regarding a drug product shall be established and followed. Such procedures shall include provisions for review by the quality control unit, of any complaint involving the possible failure of a drug product to meet any of its specifications and, for such drug products, a determination as to the need for an investigation in accordance with 211.192. Such procedures shall include provisions for review to determine whether the complaint represents a serious and unexpected adverse drug experience which is required to be reported to the Food and Drug Administration in accordance with 310.305 and 514.80 of this chapter.

(b) A written record of each complaint shall be maintained in a file designated for drug product complaints. The file regarding such drug product complaints shall be maintained at the establishment where the drug product involved was manufactured, processed, or packed, or such file may be maintained at another facility if the written records in such files are readily available for inspection at that other facility. Written records involving a drug product shall be maintained until at least 1 year after the expiration date of the drug product, or 1 year after the date that the complaint was received, whichever is longer. In the case of certain OTC drug products lacking expiration dating because they meet the criteria for exemption under 211.137, such written records shall be maintained for 3 years after distribution of the drug product.

(1) The written record shall include the following information, where known: the name and strength of the drug product, lot number, name of complainant, nature of complaint, and reply to complainant.

(2) Where an investigation under 211.192 is conducted, the written record shall include the findings of the investigation and followup. The record or copy of the record of the investigation shall be maintained at the establishment where the investigation occurred in accordance with 211.180(c).

(3) Where an investigation under 211.192 is not conducted, the written record shall include the reason that an investigation was found not to be necessary and the name of the responsible person making such a determination.

[43 FR 45077, Sept. 29, 1978, as amended at 51 FR 24479, July 3, 1986; 68 FR 15364, Mar. 31, 2003]

Subpart K--Returned and Salvaged Drug Products

Sec. 211.204 Returned drug products.

Returned drug products shall be identified as such and held. If the conditions under which returned drug products have been held, stored, or shipped before or during their return, or if the condition of the drug product, its container, carton, or labeling, as a result of storage or shipping, casts doubt on the safety, identity, strength, quality or purity of the drug product, the returned drug product shall be destroyed unless examination, testing, or other investigations prove the drug product meets appropriate standards of safety, identity, strength, quality, or purity. A drug product may be reprocessed provided the subsequent drug product meets appropriate standards, specifications, and characteristics. Records of returned drug products shall be maintained and shall include the name and label potency of the drug product dosage form, lot number (or control number or batch number), reason for the return, quantity returned, date of disposition, and ultimate disposition of the returned drug product. If the reason for a drug product being returned implicates associated batches, an appropriate investigation shall be conducted in accordance with the requirements of

211.192. Procedures for the holding, testing, and reprocessing of returned drug products shall be in writing and shall be followed.

Sec. 211.208 Drug product salvaging.

Drug products that have been subjected to improper storage conditions including extremes in temperature, humidity, smoke, fumes, pressure, age, or radiation due to natural disasters, fires, accidents, or equipment failures shall not be salvaged and returned to the marketplace. Whenever there is a question whether drug products have been subjected to such conditions, salvaging operations may be conducted only if there is (a) evidence from laboratory tests and assays (including animal feeding studies where applicable) that the drug products meet all applicable standards of identity, strength, quality, and purity and (b) evidence from inspection of the premises that the drug products and their associated packaging were not subjected to improper storage conditions as a result of the disaster or accident. Organoleptic examinations shall be acceptable only as supplemental evidence that the drug products meet appropriate standards of identity, strength, quality, and purity. Records including name, lot number, and disposition shall be maintained for drug products subject to this section.

APPENDIX II

CERTIFIED MAIL
RETURN RECEIPT REQUESTED

August 25, 2010

Mr. Jitendra Doshi
Board of Directors
Sun Pharmaceutical Industries, Inc.
270 Prospect Plains Road
Cranbury, New Jersey 08512

Dear Mr. Doshi:

During our February 25 - April 28, 2010 inspection of your pharmaceutical manufacturing facility Sun Pharmaceutical Industries, Inc., located at 270 Prospect Plains Road, Cranbury, NJ, investigators from the Food and Drug Administration (FDA) identified significant violations of Current Good Manufacturing Practice (CGMP) regulations for Finished Pharmaceuticals, Title 21, Code of Federal Regulations, Parts 210 and 211. These violations cause your drug products to be adulterated within the meaning of section 501(a)(2)(B) of the Federal Food, Drug, and Cosmetic Act (the Act) [21 U.S.C. § 351(a)(2)(B)], in that the methods used in, or the facilities or controls used for, their manufacture, processing, packing, or holding do not conform to or are not operated or administered in conformity with, CGMP.

We reviewed your firm's response of May 18, 2010, and note that it lacks sufficient corrective actions.

Specific violations observed during the inspection include, but are not limited, to the following:

1. Your firm does not have adequate written procedures for production and process controls designed to assure that the drug products you manufacture have the identity, strength, quality, and purity they purport or are represented to possess [21 C.F.R. § 211.100(a)].

For example, your firm's process for manufacturing Gernfibrozil Tablets, 600 mg, is not in a state of control and is not capable of producing batches of consistent quality. Tablets in three scale-up validation batches (90076, 90077, 90092) and three batches (BV90105, BV90111, and BV90112) made subsequent to your initial assessment of process performance, experienced "sticking and picking" defects during compression and packaging. Your firm partially released batches 90076, 90077, 90092, after culling tablets with defects, and held the other three batches. Similar defects were not observed in the two exhibit batches (70001 and 70002) manufactured in March 2007 using Magnesium Stearate supplied by (b)(4). However, the Magnesium Stearate used to manufacture the validation batches and subsequent commercial batches was supplied by (b)(4). Your January 27, 2010 initial audit of (b)(4) noted significant deficiencies which in part resulted in your change back to as (b)(4) your supplier.

In addition, initial validation batches 90031, 90032, and 90033 exhibited out-of-specification (OOS) results for unknown impurities at the six-month and nine-month room temperature stability time points. Furthermore retain samples from fifteen lots, seven of which were from initial validation batches, imploded while stored in your retain sample room.

Your response states that you will not manufacture Gemfibrozil Tablets, 600 mg, until you investigate the root cause of the impurities and imploding bottles and until you re-evaluate and revalidate the manufacturing process and all analytical methods. Before you resume manufacturing, please provide us the results of your completed investigations and documentation that demonstrates your manufacturing process is reproducible.

*We acknowledge that your firm initiated a recall of Gemfibrozil Tablets, 600 mg, on March 31, 2010, and submitted a **(b) (4)**. However, your corrective actions are inadequate. Specifically, you failed to also provide your plans to ensure the quality of distributed drug products that you manufactured using **(b)(4)** Magnesium Stearate. In addition, you failed to provide your plans to ensure that the ingredient suppliers for all of your drug products are adequately qualified.*

2. Your firm has not thoroughly investigated the failure of a batch or any of its components to meet its specifications, whether or not the batch has already been distributed, or extended investigations to other batches of drug product that may have been associated with the specific failure or discrepancy [21 C.F.R. § 211.192]. For example,

> *a. Although your firm was aware of imploding bottles of Gemfibrozil Tablets, 600mg, in September 2009, you did not initiate a root-cause investigation or conduct a recall to the retail level until our inspection. The retain samples from fifteen lots of Gemfibrozil Tablets, 600 mg, imploded while in your retain sample room. You distributed the lots from March 25, 2009, to June 24, 2009.*

Your response is inadequate in that you did not explain why you failed to open an investigation in September 2009, when you first identified the problem. Timely assessment of quality indicators, such as OOS findings and complaints, is essential to detecting and determining the scope of product or process deficiencies. In response to this observation, please also provide the details of the investigation and the suspected root cause.

> *b. During release testing, batches 90056 and 90057 of Promethazine Hydrochloride (HCl) Tablets, 25 mg, exhibited OOS water content results of 5.7% and 5.9%, respectively (the specification is **(b)(4)**). The OOS results were invalidated after a retest yielded acceptable results, despite your failure to identify an assignable laboratory cause. Furthermore, you failed to extend the investigation to associated batches. The investigation did not include batch 90058 that was analyzed*

in conjunction with batches 90056 and 90057 and for which passing results were obtained. Yet your Quality Control Unit (QCU) released lots 90056A, 90057A, and 90058A between May 2009 and June 2009.

Your response states that: 1) **(b)(4)** *will review all current OOS investigations to determine their adequacy; 2) you will revise Standard Operating Procedure (SOP) 2.2.43, "Handling Out-of-Specification Results," to be consistent with FDA guidance "Investigating Out-of-Specification (OOS) Test Results for Pharmaceutical Production;" and 3) you will revise OOS worksheets to ensure consistency with SOP 2.2.43. We cannot evaluate the adequacy of your response because you have not completed the investigation and have not implemented most of your proposed corrective actions. In your response, please clarify whether review will include investigations from the previous two years and future investigations.*

3. Your firm has failed to ensure the responsibilities and procedures applicable to your quality control unit are followed [21 C.F.R. § 211.22(d)]. For example,

a. The QCU failed to ensure customer complaints were adequately investigated as required by SOP 1.1.16, "Quality Unit," dated November 12, 2007. Between August 27, 2008, and December 16, 2009, you received fourteen complaints of leaking capsules for multiple lots of Nimodipine Capsules, 30 mg. Your "Corrective Action Summary for Nimodipine Capsules, 30 mg," signed by the Quality Assurance Manager on October 8, 2009, states your firm and your contract manufacturer, **(b) (4)** *thoroughly investigated the complaints. The investigation determined that the potency results for the leaking capsules met specifications. However, your November 11-12, 2009 audit of* **(b)(4)** *concluded that* **(b)(4)** *failed to properly determine the impact of product efficacy. Your corrective action summary also identifies the root cause of the leaking capsules and describes the changes made to the formulation, capsule shell, capsule fill weight, and equipment processing parameters based on "small scale experiments." Your QCU approved these changes without* *verifying the revalidation of the affected manufacturing processes to ensure that the changes were effective and did not adversely affect the drug product.*

Your response states you will revise your Quality Agreement with to (b)(4) clarify how you will handle investigations and you consider your "enhanced process" to be validated. Your response is inadequate because you failed to provide documentation to support your conclusion that the process is validated. You also failed to provide scientific justification for allowing Nimodipine Capsule lots made prior to the changes to remain on the market.

b. Your QCU failed to adequately review production and control records to ensure no errors occurred, as required by your SOP 1.1.16. Our investigators noted a discrepancy in the analytical records related to the finished product testing of lot 90056, Promethazine HCl Tablets, 25 mg. The analytical records indicate that you tested lot 80056, rather than lot 90056, for assay. Yet your QCU approved and released lot 90056 without noting the discrepancy.

Your response states that analyst transcription error caused the discrepancy and that the lot was properly assayed prior to release. You state that your firm initiated investigation IR 10-006 to determine why the transcription error was not identified prior to release and the appropriate corrective and preventative action plan. However, we cannot determine the adequacy of your response because you failed to provide us with your completed investigation, IR 10-006.

c. Your QCU failed to follow SOP 1.1.14, "Product Recall Procedure," dated May 26, 2006, by failing to notify the FDA when you recalled multiple lots of Gemfibrozil Tablets, 600 mg, on October 23, 2009 from your distributor (b)(4).

Your response states that although you consider (b)(4) warehouse an extension of Sun's warehouse, an SOP will be created to define the control mechanisms for product manufactured at Sun and distributed by (b)(4). We cannot determine the adequacy of your response because you failed to provide any further details which demonstrate that the affected Gemfibrozil lots were not recalled because they hadn't left Sun's direct control.

4. Your firm does not adequately inspect the packaging and labeling facilities immediately before use to assure that all drug products have been removed from the previous operations [21 C.F.R. § 211.130(e)].

For example, on July 14, 2009, you found four Oxycodone HCI Tablets, 5 mg, in the brushes of Packaging Line (b)(4) while packaging Oxycodone HCI Tablets, 15 mg, lot 90088A. The 5 mg tablets were from lot 90087A which was packaged on line (b)(4) between July 7 and 10, 2009. Although you cleaned and inspected the line before packaging lot 90088A, you failed to detect the 5 mg tablets from lot 90087A. In addition, your investigation, IR 09-106, failed to determine the adequacy of your line clearance procedures and the need for improvements.

Your response states that you consider a line clearance failure to be a critical issue and that you are drafting a new SOP to ensure adequate packaging line clearance. However, we cannot evaluate the adequacy of your response because you failed to provide this SOP. Your response also states that you evaluated the impact of this incident on previously packaged products. In your response, please provide further details regarding this evaluation.

5. Your firm has not established and followed written procedures prescribing a system for reprocessing batches that do not conform to standards or specifications and the steps taken to insure that the reprocessed batches will conform with all established standards, specifications, and characteristics [21 C.F.R. § 211.115(a)], nor does your firm perform reprocessing with the review and approval of the quality control unit [21 C.F.R. § 211.115(b)].

For example, during the packaging of Gemfibrozil Tablets, 600 mg, lot 90076A, on August 6, 2009, you emptied under-filled bottles into the hopper for repackaging without an approved written procedure and without the approval of the QCU.

Your response acknowledges that you conducted "non-quality related reprocessing operations" without QCU approval and that an impact assessment was performed. Your response also states that packaging operations ceased on March 25, 2010, and will not resume until appropriate corrective actions are implemented. We cannot assess the adequacy of your response because you have not provided any documentation such as your impact assessment, revised packaging procedure, and enhancements to your Quality System to ensure similar deviations are identified during the Quality Unit's review of production records.

In addition, our inspection revealed that you failed to submit NDA Field Alert Reports to FDA in compliance with 21 C.F.R. § 314.81(b)(1)(ii), as required by section 505(k) of the Act [21 U.S.C. § 355(k)]. 21 C.F.R. § 314.81(b)(1)(ii) requires an applicant to submit information within three working days of date of discovery concerning any bacteriological contamination, or any significant chemical, physical, or other change or deterioration in the distributed drug product, or any failure of one or more distributed batches of drug product to meet the specifications established for it in the application. Specifically:

> *a. On September 30,2009, multiple lots of Gemfibrozil Tablets, 600 mg, 500 and 1000 count were noted by your Quality Unit to have imploded in the sample room. After noting this physical deterioration, Gemfibrozil Tablets, 500 count, were distributed into interstate commerce from March 25, 2009 through September 1, 2009. No Field Alert Report was filed for this incident.*

> *b. From September 8, 2008, to December 16, 2009, fourteen consumer complaints of leaking and sweating Nimodipine Capsules, 30 mg, were received. After assessment by your QCU, a corrective action plan was implemented which included changes to your drug product formulation and soft gelatin capsule shell. These changes took place in June 2009. A Field Alert Report was not reported until March 15, 2010, when FDA conducted an inspection of your facility.*

c. From May 19, 2009, to January 13, 2010, five complaints of two lots of Oxycodone Tablets, 5 mg and 30 mg (lots 90072 and 90069A) were received. Complaints ranged from under-filled bottles to a missing bottle in a packaging shipper. Because Oxycodone is a controlled substance (Schedule II) under the Controlled Substance Act [21 U.S.C. § 801 et seq.], all tablets should be accounted and reconciled. An NDA/ANDA Field Alert Report was provided on March 24, 2010, when FDA conducted an inspection of your facility.

Your response is inadequate because your corrective actions to address Field Alert Reporting do not comply with the requirement of 21 C.F.R. § 314.81. Your response indicates your complaint handling procedures will be revised to prevent recurrence of the drug product quality defects; however no details of your revised procedures were provided.

The violations cited in this letter are not intended to be an all inclusive list of violations that may exist at your facility. You are responsible for investigating and determining the causes of the violations identified above and for preventing their recurrence and the occurrence of other violations. It is your responsibility to assure compliance with all requirements of federal law and FDA regulations.

You should take prompt action to correct the violations cited in this letter. Failure to promptly correct these violations may result in legal action without further notice including, without limitation, seizure and injunction. Other federal agencies may take this Warning Letter into account when considering the award of contracts. Additionally, FDA may withhold approval of requests for export certificates, or approval of new drug applications listing your facilities, until the above violations are corrected. FDA may re-inspect to verify corrective actions have been completed.

Within fifteen (15) working days of receipt of this letter, please notify this office in writing of the specific steps you have taken to correct violations. Include an explanation of each step taken to prevent the recurrence of violations and copies of supporting documentation. If you cannot complete corrective action within fifteen working days, state the reason for the delay and the date by which you will have completed the correction. Additionally, your response should state if you no longer manufacture or distribute the drug products manufactured at these facilities, and provide the date(s) and reason(s) you ceased production.

Your response should be addressed to: U.S. Food and Drug Administration, 10 Waterview Boulevard, 3rd Floor, Parsippany, New Jersey, 07054, Attn: Sarah A. Della Fave, Compliance Officer.

Sincerely,

/s/

Diana Amador-Toro
District
Director
New Jersey District

www.ingramcontent.com/pod-product-compliance
Lightning Source LLC
Chambersburg PA
CBHW030318290526
45785CB00001B/416